Advance Praise for Catt Tripoli's *Conscious Fitness* . . .

The title of this marvelous book says it all: CONSCIOUS . . . FITNESS go hand in glove. In doing the sports we love, we have all suspected a larger dimension, which includes body, mind, emotion, soul and Spirit. Catt Tripoli, body builder, champion athlete, has put it together for us in this exceptional, practical, go-out-and-do-it book.

– **David Meggyesy,** Former NFL linebacker,
Author: *Out of Their League*

After 40 years, my weight-lifting training has been transformed. *Conscious Fitness* provides superb foundational knowledge in physiology, anatomy and appreciation of the marvelous human body for your physical training, and adds the gift of taking her knowledge from her practice in wisdom traditions to craft her performance-changing consciousness practices for consistent top results.

– **Greg Warburton,** MS, Author: *Warburton's Winning System: Tapping and Other Transformational Mental Training Tools for Athletes*

As a successful health studio owner operator, champion women's bodybuilding competitor, and life long fitness advocate, Catt Tripoli comes well qualified to write her new book *Conscious Fitness: Strength Training for the Evolution of Body, Mind, and Spirit*. She draws upon her life experiences well, giving practical advice enabling others to avoid much of the trial and error that accompanies physical, mental, and spiritual growth. Not only is it a book for those beginning weight training, it's also useful for those who are already training because it's full of gems.

– **Frank Zane,** M.A., Mr. America, Mr. World,
3-Time Mr. Universe, 3-Time Mr. Olympia
www.frankzane.com

Catt Tripoli weaves together personal stories, explorations into Native American wisdom and the use of hypnotherapy to access the power of mind, all illustrating the amazing creative potential we can all access. *Conscious Fitness* is powerfully motivating, inspiring and full of wisdom.

– **Cheryl Canfield,** author of *Profound Healing.*

Catt Tripoli's dramatic personal journey would in itself make for a fascinating book. But she takes us far beyond her own story, sharing with us her profound insights into what it means to be truly fit, as well as the vital knowledge that mind, body, and spirit are one.

– **Lyn 'Unihipiliowailelepualu Moreno,**
traditional healer, teacher of The Path of Aloha,
and instructor at Hypnotherapy Training Institute

Conscious Fitness

Conscious Fitness

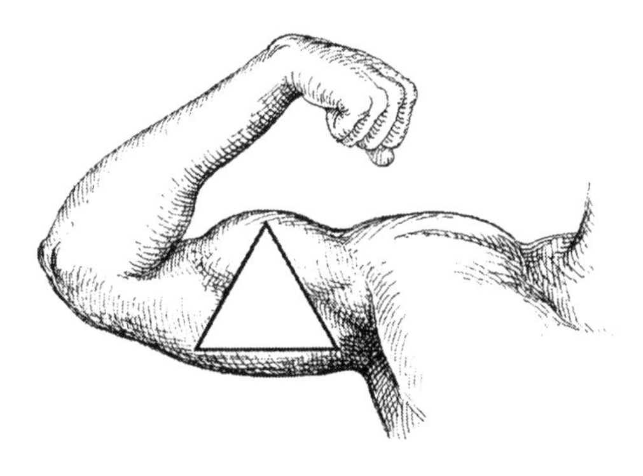

Strength Training for the Evolution of Body, Mind, and Spirit

CATT TRIPOLI *with JoAnne O'Brien-Levin*

Illustrations by Michael Bergt

Bull Terrier Publishing • Santa Rosa, California

First Edition

Published by Bull Terrier Publishing
Santa Rosa, California
www.phgsr.com

ISBN 978-0-692-67572-4

Editor and writer: JoAnne O'Brien-Levin
Illustrations by Michael Bergt
Cover and book design by Ann Lowe
Anatomy illustrations from www.123rf.com
Printed by CreateSpace
Typeface: Univers and Chaparral Pro

This book is dedicated to all my teachers –
both intentional and accidental.
You helped make this work possible.

Acknowledgments

A VERY SPECIAL THANK YOU to my friend and editor, Joanne O'Brien-Levin, who pushed, pulled, prodded, cajoled, threatened and ultimately brought my words to life. I cannot thank you enough.

And to my Best Friend, Sammie Freitag-Batten, I am so grateful to have found you again after 25 years! Had I not undertaken the writing of this book, and had Joanne O'Brien-Levin not been a better sleuth than I, we would have remained lost to each other. I am forever grateful to Spirit for the synchronicities that moved this project forward and that helped me find you – and that the will of the cult, ultimately, was not stronger than the loving bond we have.

To my mentor, Tu Moonwalker – thank you for putting me on the path and waking me up. I continue to miss your presence.

Thanks to Dave Weeks for introducing me to the iron. It changed everything.

Thanks to Bill Palyo for giving me the encouragement to compete and the support I needed to train, compete and win.

Thank you to Michael Bergt and Steve Aja who so graciously offered up their respective, amazing talents for this "little" project.

To my cousin David, whom I found after 45 years, during the course of writing this book. Thank you for believing in me and this project.

Thank you to my "tribe" – Beth Ghashghai, and Laurie and Mike Dillabough for being the best cheerleading section, EVER!

And finally, thank you to everyone and everything that has risen up to support my being every day. No one lives their life in a vacuum, my surviving and THRIVING depends on the altruism of the Universe. I am eternally grateful.

And finally, thank you to my father, Guiseppe Patrick Enrico Tripoli, for making me an insane perfectionist with an eye for the minutest structural abnormality. And to my mother, Dorothy Muriel Tripoli (nee Magnano) for knowing about the importance of nutrition, long before it was fashionable. They both did the best they knew how, with the tools that were in their toolbox.

TABLE OF CONTENTS

Introduction

WITH THIS BOOK, I hope to change your concept of fitness. Fitness is *not only about the body*. It's not just about the exercises we do (or don't do). It's about the way we go about working out, whether we do so consciously or by rote. True fitness begins before we ever touch a piece of equipment, and it's about how present we are while we're working out.

You see, in many respects, the real gym is within.

Conscious Fitness is your guidebook for mastering that inner territory and applying that knowledge to maximize your bodybuilding workout. I know the term "bodybuilding" can put some people off, so I want to be clear: there's a big distinction between bodybuilding in general, and *competitive* bodybuilding. **If you're working out in order to strengthen your muscles and re-shape your body, you *are* bodybuilding,** and you would benefit from learning the skills and techniques I've learned from being a world champion competitive bodybuilder and from training regular people for multiple decades.

In this book, I explain why consciousness is the hidden key to transforming your workout—why it not only makes your workout more efficient, but also catalyzes re-connection at the deepest levels of your being.

Therefore, this is not simply a book about physical fitness—though there's plenty of information about that—it's also a book about becoming more conscious and attuned to the interrelationship between our bodies and our minds and spirits.

Conscious Fitness empowers people to inhabit their bodies fully; it's about taking back your power by tuning into yourself. Conscious Fitness is about becoming strong in an age that promotes comfort and fosters excess. Committing to be fit is, in and of itself, an act of courage, even insurrection, because so much about our culture strives to keep us soft, weak, inattentive—and unconscious.

The way we approach fitness is equally important. The images in magazines can make us feel inadequate; we can be tempted to over-do to achieve some ideal of perfection. But that, too, is a symptom of our lack of consciousness. Fitness needs to *fit* into our lives in a balanced way. Conscious Fitness is not about becoming "shredded," or making every workout epic; it's about consistent, conscious practice. It's about making oneself strong and whole, one muscle, one exercise, one day at a time.

The approach described in *Conscious Fitness* comes out of my 36 years of study, my practice and experience in the world of fitness as a world champion female bodybuilder, personal trainer and gym owner. It draws from sources as diverse as ballet, hypnosis, Western science and Native wisdom.

By making my *Conscious Fitness* approach accessible to all I hope to encourage everyone who reads it to discover a new level of self-empowerment. I'm convinced that, no matter what your path, developing a strong body is key to your becoming the best you can be. I know it can give you the foundation you need to pursue your dreams. I'm writing this book in order to present that case to you, and to offer you my ideas—based on my experience—for how to create your own best, strong body.

As you read *Conscious Fitness,* you'll develop a more intimate connection with your *body.* You'll come to appreciate the *mind's* role in fitness, and witness the rewards when you shift from distraction to focus. You'll discover a *spiritual* dimension to fitness, *i.e.*, how lifting weights can lift your spirit by helping you transcend traumas and self-imposed limits.

Conscious Fitness is also about falling in love with real, nourishing food and becoming more attentive to our diets. Proper nutrition is an essential support to our wellbeing; it is also a source of vitality and joy.

If you adopt my *Conscious Fitness* approach you will see your workout—and fitness in general—in a whole new way. Practically speaking, you'll be more inspired to work out, and you'll feel more empowered to take creative control of your workout (and your life). You'll be able to maximize your time in the gym, while also protecting yourself from injury. As a consequence, you'll see and feel results. My techniques will make you stronger and more powerful—not only physically, but also mentally and spiritually. You'll feel more energized, integrated, and whole, both within and without. You'll become more capable of setting—and achieving—the fitness goals that are right for you. And, by achieving what you set out to do, you'll raise the bar on yourself. You'll stop seeing yourself as a product of your limiting beliefs, and start seeing yourself as you really are: an open field of possibility: a shape shifter.

The book begins by laying the philosophical groundwork of its premise. Separate chapters are devoted to helping you get reacquainted with your body, mind and spirit and their relationship to Conscious Fitness. The book then makes the case for strength training—working with weights—as essential to fitness, especially as we age, and describes the three main types of strength training.

It follows by describing the essential aspects of the *Conscious Fitness* approach. I describe a step-by-step approach to help you master the inner art of working with weights so that you can maximize effectiveness and avoid injury. The Conscious Fitness approach to dealing with discomfort and pain is also discussed.

The book concludes with a wealth of practical information designed to empower readers to take control of their workouts and optimize their gym experience. For example, I discuss why it is so important to avoid fitness "routines," because this is the very antithesis of consciousness; it's another way give up control and go on autopilot. I give you tools to help you design *your* workout.

Along the way, I'll share aspects of my personal story—not because I'm so special, but because I'm average in so many ways, with many of the same insecurities and doubts that plague us all. I hope my story will act as a kind of mirror. Through it, I hope you'll see your own reflection and that it will help you to find your own road to fitness, health, and wellbeing.

Here's an outline of the book, chapter by chapter:

Introduction: Here, I introduce you to my Conscious Fitness approach.

Chapter 1, Conscious Fitness: The Essential Triangle: In this chapter I explain how—and why—we achieve optimal fitness through the integration of body, mind, and spirit. I follow with chapters dedicated to a greater understanding of our bodies, our minds, and our spirits.

Chapter 2, My Journey to Conscious Fitness: My Conscious Fitness approach is based on the idea that optimal fitness and wellbeing comes through integrating our bodies, minds and spirits. Here, I establish my credentials by providing some background about my journey and how I developed my approach. By revealing the many obstacles, both inner and outer, that I faced and transcended through the greater integration of Body-Mind-Spirit, I hope to establish myself as a relate-able role model and source of inspiration for others.

Chapter 3, Body: An Intimate Journey: Most of us are disconnected from our bodies. We're so disconnected that we've contracted out the care of our bodies, turning them over the pharmaceutical and medical communities. But medicine is a business, as is Big Pharma; they may have the ability to tell us what to do when we're sick, but they have no incentive to help us be well. Everything else is collateral damage. In this chapter I encourage you to re-connect with—even fall in love with—the miracle that is your body. I also provide a guided tour of your major muscle groups that you can use to help you visualize during your workout.

Chapter 4, Getting your Mind in Shape: Our minds can be our greatest allies—or our enemies and saboteurs. In this chapter I discuss how to get our minds aligned so they support our efforts to become fit.

Chapter 5, The Spirit of Fitness: Yes, there is a spiritual aspect to fitness. In this chapter I explore the connection.

Chapter 6, The Case for Weight Training: This chapter explains why strength training, *i.e.*, working with weights, is so essential to fitness.

Chapter 7, Three Kinds of Weight Training: This chapter gives you a basic overview of three different styles of strength training: power lifting, conditioning, and bodybuilding. It explains the purpose, strengths and downsides of each so that you can choose intelligently. It also explains why my Conscious Fitness approach, which derives from my experience with bodybuilding, provides a solid foundational, whichever path you choose.

Chapter 8, The Heart of the Technique: This chapter introduces the major principles that underlie my Conscious Fitness approach: muscle isolation and opposition.

Chapter 9, Conscious Fitness Step-by-Step, Part 1: Preparation: In this chapter and the next I take you on a step-by-step guided tour of how to apply my Conscious Fitness approach to your workout. This chapter explains eight steps you can use to help integrate your mind, body and spirit for an optimal workout. Following these practices—which only takes moments—will help *bring more consciousness* into your workout, thus maximizing benefit.

Chapter 10, Conscious Fitness Step-by-Step, Part 2: Lifting Consciously: Continuing from the previous chapter, this chapter focuses on lifting and describes seven additional aspects of the "the gym within." Among other things, you'll learn the Conscious Fitness approach to working with weights and also how to respond consciously to discomfort or pain.

Chapter 11, Workout Wisdom: Empowering You to Take Control of Your Workout: I don't advocate exercise "routines" as they aren't really efficient, and the very idea of following a routine is antithetical to my conscious approach. In this chapter I empower readers with the knowledge they need to design their own "non-routine routines" so that they can execute workouts that have maximum impact on their health and wellbeing.

Chapter 12, Food: A Love Story: Proper nourishment is key to health and wellbeing. This chapter is intended to inspire readers to fall in love with good, healthy food and to show them how taking a more conscious approach to meal planning, grocery shopping and meal preparation can transform their lives.

Appendix: What You Need to Own your Workout – Tips, Pointers, & FAQs: This is grab bag of information that will make you more knowledgeable and feel more empowered in the gym.

1. Conscious Fitness

THE ESSENTIAL TRIANGLE

CONSCIOUS FITNESS actually redefines our understanding of fitness. As I said, fitness is not just about the body; it is about *the integration of Body-Mind-Spirit.*

Body-Mind-Spirit integration is extremely important because it is the source of true power. The more integrated we are, the more powerful we are. However, our Body, Mind and Spirit don't harmonize without conscious effort; that's why we often feel fragmented, distracted and dis-integrated. My Conscious Fitness approach is a way to bring about that integration, leading to a surge in positive energy, vitality, and wellbeing. We achieve this integration by taking a *conscious* approach to our workouts.

Conscious Fitness is about becoming more attuned to our *bodies*—how they work and how they are supposed to *feel*, in a deep, not superficial way. In a world full of noise, this is a book about turning inward to listen to one's body, to one's inner voice, to one's deeper wisdom. As I've learned, our bodies are great allies and great teachers. Through our bodies, by testing them and asking things of them, we learn who we are.

It's about becoming more aware of how our *minds* work and how our mental habits can sabotage our commitment to fitness. It's also about how we can harness our mind's innate power to commune with our bodies, our musculature, all our parts, and achieve results we never thought possible.

Spirit, I know, is a controversial topic. What place does it have in a gym? I believe *fitness has a spiritual dimension*, and that I may be uniquely qualified to bring that to light in a balanced way because of my background. I was raised in a very dogmatic belief system—some might call it a cult. My early experience with this system, which I rebelled against, caused me to have great skepticism about spiritual matters for many years. In time, though, I came to recognize spirit as an essential part of our being, an aspect we just can't ignore. I'll speak about that in more depth in later chapters.

My Conscious Fitness approach brings together three things that are often considered very separate—as if they have nothing to do with one another: body, mind and spirit.

As I've said, fitness is not just about the body. Yet, because we tend to think that it is *only* about the body, we can go on "autopilot" during our workouts; we can fill them with distractions, such as music and television. But when we do that, when we don't really connect to what we're doing and just go through the motions, we're not *present*. These workouts are "unconscious." Unconscious workouts have some benefit, of course, but much less than they could. Further, they reinforce a fallacy central to modern our lives: that our bodies are separate from our minds, from our spirits. This belief harms us in innumerable ways, creating disharmony and disintegration both within and without.

Conscious Fitness, on the other hand, recognizes the importance of creating and maintaining an intimate interconnection between our bodies, our minds, and our spirits. That relationship is essential for our wellbeing. Here's why:

Many say we have seven chakras, or energy centers, each of which vibrates at a different frequency. In the chakra system the frequencies go from lowest (the root chakra), to highest (crown chakra). The role of the chakra system is to take in vital energy from the environment and transform it into the frequencies needed by the various areas of our physical bodies for maintenance and development.

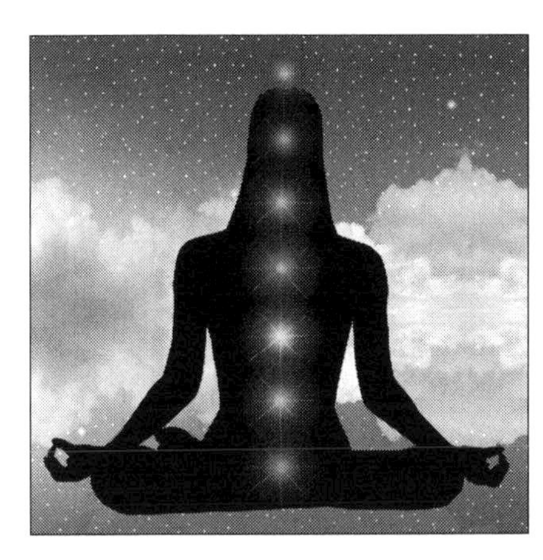

CROWN

THIRD EYE

THROAT

HEART

SOLAR PLEXUS

SACRAL

ROOT

This is not just "New Age" fantasy. Quantum physics also tells us that everything is energy; even things appearing to be rock-solid are just dense forms of energy. And energy is always in motion. Vibration is the essence of the universe, and everything vibrates at a different frequency.

This has a bearing on our health and wellbeing. Our bodies, minds, and spirits are very different in their nature, and they naturally vibrate at different frequencies. But these frequencies can *harmonize*. When we are in a state of health, these vibrations harmonize in a way that makes us *radiant*; our wellbeing is palpable to others.

However, entropy is a law of the Universe. Everything tends toward disorganization and deterioration: things fall apart; we age; ongoing maintenance is required. This is true of the integration of our Body-Mind-Spirit as well; they tend to fall out of harmony with each other. We can allow—even mindlessly *enable*—that disintegration, or we can work actively toward integration, toward more *wholeness*, on an ongoing basis. The wisdom of this is actually embedded in our language: the words "health," "wholeness" and even "holy" derive from the same root in Old English.[1]

Exercise, done *consciously*, is a means to that integration. A conscious workout involves not just our bodies, but includes our minds and spirits as well. When we bring all three into our workouts, *our workouts are not just more efficient; they're transformative*—on multiple levels.

Let's look at these three aspects of our wholeness in a bit more depth:

Body

I see the body as the vessel that houses our mind and spirit, enabling us to move, interact and interface with everything in our environment. It's also our first line of defense. The physical body is foundational structure for everything else. No edifice is stable if its foundation is not rock-solid. So, the body's health and wellbeing are essential to the thriving of our mental and spiritual lives. This is why we have to take care of our bodies.

Because our physical body is denser than our mind or spirit, it vibrates at a slower frequency than these. This is natural. If, however, we ingest unhealthy food, water or other liquids that are polluted with toxins, and we don't exercise on a consistent basis, we actually slow our body's vibration below what's natural or optimal. This makes it harder to achieve integration with our other, less dense parts—mind and spirit—that vibrate at a higher frequency naturally. In short, we begin to dis-integrate. We have to maintain the body's natural vibration so that we can be in a state of wholeness, a state of health.

Conscious fitness asks you to become intimately connected with your own physical being, to build a relationship with it, to commune and commiserate with it. It advocates connecting your body with your mind and spirit.

Mind

Conscious fitness is a workout philosophy that details how to manage yourself and your mind so you can be a healthier, happier person. It's a way of *shaping the body by focusing the mind*, a skill I learned and continued to hone through my study of hypnosis. You see, the mind and the body are meant to work together; when they do, we experience a real sense of power. But, too often, we have them doing separate things. The body is exercising, but the mind is distracted by a TV screen or by music playing through our earphones—or it's just wandering. When we distract ourselves, we siphon energy away from our workout; it's an energy leak. We become fragmented—not whole—and thus, we're not moving toward health. But when you bring your focused mind into the equation, your workout improves exponentially. Your mind and your body become a team, working together to shape and re-shape your body in accordance with your intention.

Conscious Fitness advocates connecting your body and mind (and spirit). You create that connection by tuning into your body, consciously attending to it with your mind, not distracting yourself from what it's doing.

When you have a completely focused mind, everything else drops away. All your energy is laser-focused toward achieving a singular goal. There's just you and your workout. It's an absolutely delicious feeling. In addition, you have a different relationship to discomfort and pain. Pain, which we'll also discuss in depth later in this book, is a fundamental part of the workout process. We tend to run from it, for obvious reasons. But some pain is necessary if we are to make progress. Yes, the phrase "No pain, no gain" is true, but I'm not talking about over-doing it. I can't emphasize this enough: I'm not talking about going to extremes, and I'm absolutely not advocating your putting yourself in danger. No, I'm talking about that minimal amount of pain that's needed to signal that you're crossing a threshold: that a muscle is breaking down in order to re-build. It's the necessary price to make you stronger.

When your mind and body are out of synch, disconnected, you'll tend to react to that pain threshold *mindlessly*. You'll bail out too early and thus lose out on the benefit. But when your mind and body are in tune, you can work with pain in a much more controlled way, which is ultimately safer and way more productive. It's much more efficient—in terms of both time and energy—than running from pain, which actually makes us more exhausted.

Spirit

Most of us have been conditioned to see the body as separate from spirit, but I see the two as intimately connected. Despite my early experiences with a dogmatic belief system, I've learned to accept the idea that there is something beyond the physical or material plane. It seems self-evident to me that there's something that animates us, something that gives the flesh life, that makes us who we are. As humans, we may never understand exactly what spirit is, but that doesn't mean we have to ignore its existence.

I believe that means you have to have some consciousness about your physical being in order to be able to attain a higher level of spiritual awareness. How can we build a strong ethereal body if we don't begin with the physical? This body is what we have to move our spirit through the world, so if we ignore or abuse it, we're harming our connection to spirit. And we can abuse our bodies by not being fit.

I hope you can understand that I'm not advocating any religious beliefs, per se; I'm just acknowledging the existence of something beyond us that we can call spirit.

Conscious Fitness integrates the physical with the mental and, in so doing, connects us with the level of existence we know as spirit. It's about using our minds to develop our muscles. It's about directing energy (which may be another word for "spirit"). To explain this connection further, I'd like to share a little about my life and how I came to this understanding.

Roots: Native Wisdom

Ever since I can remember, I've had an affinity for Native American culture, especially because of the strong connection to nature and the Earth that underlies these ways. Why this affinity is so deep, I don't know, but it seems to go back to my birth.

I was born in the Emergency Room in the hospital in Big Bear, California. As I heard the story told by my parents, there was still snow on ground—not unusual for the mountains in March--and I was coming fast. My father put my mother in the car and sped to the hospital over icy roads, arriving just before I came into the world. The hospital didn't have time to get my mother into a room, so they just put her in one of those bays in the ER.

Big Bear is ski country, and all around my mother, ER doctors were hard at work treating the sprained ankles and broken legs of the patrons of the nearby ski resort. My mother said there was just a curtain separating her and the team setting someone's leg, so she could hear everything and, more importantly I suppose, so could they. To add to the festivities, my father was present at my birth. In those days, that was quite unusual. He witnessed my birth, though he may not have wanted to! (He later described it as pretty stressful.) But when he first laid eyes on me what struck him was that I had this long, blue-black hair. He said if he hadn't seen the birth himself, he would have sworn the hospital had given them the wrong infant because I looked like a Native American baby. From that day forward, he called me "Papoose."

That connection with native ways persisted throughout my life, like a distant calling from destiny. Always, I loved and identified with

Native American things. For example, whenever I went riding, I wore Navajo hats and moccasins instead of the cowboy hats and boots that all the other kids wore. Several times during my youth, my family traveled cross-country by car. Those trips were special because I got to see some Native cultural artifacts, such as the Anasazi cliff dwellings in Colorado. But most of all, I remember the feeling I got when we crossed the state line into New Mexico, the most indigenous state in the union. The minute we crossed the border, I felt like I could finally breathe. I didn't feel this way in Arizona or Utah, only in New Mexico. And believe me, it wasn't because of the natural beauty of the place. We were traveling on Route 66, which does not go through the best parts.

So, many years later, when a good friend, Beth, suggested that I begin studying with some Native American teachers she had worked with in New Mexico, I got goose bumps. Something about it felt very right. Even though I was deeply skeptical of most religious traditions (due to my upbringing), I very much wanted to delve into and explore spirituality from a Native American perspective. Looking back now, I don't think it was ever what I imagined it would be. It was always deeper, much deeper.

By the time I started studying with these Native teachers, Tu Moonwalker and Lané Sa'an Moonwalker, I was close to 45 years of age. I felt my approach to fitness already rested on a very solid foundation, but their teachings progressed me even further.

Their approach to spirituality made sense to me because it was so practical, so earthbound, so grounded in the experience of being "in a human suit," as they put it. Their teachings were a response to questions that reverberate in the human heart: *How can we, as humans, create a real and meaningful relationship with the Divine?* How can we create a truly *authentic* relationship with the Divine, a relationship that isn't based on illusion? What does it mean to be a human being with all its complexities and contradictions? And what obligations and responsibilities come with being human?

They were realists in a way I'd never experienced before; they saw clear through to the essence of what it means to be a human being—with all the virtues and all the flaws inherent to our species. And, without flinching, they accepted all of it, managed it, and taught their students to do the same. Having been raised in an apocryphal belief system that demanded blind allegiance, I was unendingly skeptical; I resisted dogma of any kind. But this was not that. I sensed a great deal of truth in their presentations. Their teachings resonated with my core.

The Mind-Body-Spirit Connection

In particular, they taught that the human being is not just one thing, not just one entity. We're made up of many different components: blood, muscles, bones, organs, enzymes, cells, platelets, hormonal glands, emotions, even our ancestors! All these disparate parts have their own particular needs and ways of being.

Because of this, the human being is really complex, a fact we don't tend to fully appreciate. My teachers talked about how we were made up of five different "bodies." Besides the physical body, there are the mental, the emotional, the spiritual, and the psychic bodies. Each of these relates to things in a different way. They taught us to do an exercise where we'd check in with these different aspects of ourselves by asking:

- *What am I feeling physically?*
- *Mentally?*
- *Emotionally?*
- *Spiritually?*
- *Psychically?*

Through that exercise we'd discover that we had all these different dimensions to our experience. This would help sensitize us to how multifaceted human beings really are.

These teachings validated what I'd already known instinctively. I could see so clearly now that we are a composite of all these different parts—as well as the elements of fire, water, earth and air. When I finally began to understand what they were saying, I was blown open about how complex it all is. Yet, despite this complexity, these different aspects all work together to create the wholeness of our being. In short, we are a walking, talking collaboration of all these disparate parts. What a miracle!

And what is true of the human body (the micro) is true of the Universe (the macro); all these disparate things have to come together to make it work. When I was finally able to take that in, I saw the planet in a new way, as a vast web of cooperation.

It's been said that when Magellan and his crew made their way to shore at what they called Tierra del Fuego, or "Land of the Fire," named for the many campfires built by the Indigenous people who inhabited the landscape at the southernmost tip of South America, they were astonished to find that the Native people literally could not see their huge, masted ships in the harbor. The reason was that the Indigenous people's conceptual frameworks did not include anything like those enormous, seafaring galleons. Therefore, the boats were invisible to them.[2]

This is the example of "believing is seeing," meaning we can't see what we don't already believe in. By the same token, we can't see the world as a vast web of cooperation if we're conditioned to focus on competition. We've been so conditioned to see Nature as "red in tooth and claw," as the saying goes, that we are blind to the myriad ways in which Nature is cooperative. Cooperation is part of nature, down to the cellular level. The reason why is simple, according to evolutionary biologists: Cooperation is one of the most important and beneficial behaviors on Earth. We literally would not be here without it.

Humans, plants, and animals are made up of cells that learned to cooperate long ago. They got together to form multi-cellular organisms, thereby increasing each individual cell's chances of survival—and replication—in the process. Cooperation prevails at every level of the animal kingdom, as research has pointed out. Ants collectively manage their traffic. Smaller fish rid bigger fish of harmful bacteria by swimming into their mouths; the one gets a cleaner mouth and the other, a meal. Small birds alert larger birds of predators, and get protected in the process. Bats can't live two nights without food, so bats share their food with those who are without.[3] All of this occurs for the evolution of the entire organism.

The chain of cooperation starts at the smallest level, and moves up. "From molecules joining together to form compartments at the beginning of life, through replicators joining together to form chromosomes, through prokaryotes combining to form the eukaryotes, cells multiplying into multi-cellular organisms and individuals forming colonies, cooperation is ubiquitous. We cannot chalk up its existence to a few exceptions and it must be incorporated as a building block in evolutionary theory." This was a groundbreaking insight from William D. Hamilton, one of the greats of evolutionary theory of the 1960s."[4]

This was the vision that my teachers imparted to me. And I know that whenever any species goes extinct—as so many are now—it diminishes the Whole. Like the natives of Tierra del Fuego, we may not be able to see all those connecting threads, but they're there.

Integrating Our Selves

If you think about it, these three major aspects of our selves—Mind, Body, and Spirit—are vastly different in kind and quality. I suggest you take a moment to get in touch with that idea. See if you can feel how each has a very the different kind of energy.

Sometimes it helps to think of these different aspects symbolically, as animals, for example. You might think of your body as a big cat, a mountain lion perhaps, so physical in its being; sleek, lithe and graceful; inhabiting its body fully. Or maybe it's more like a bear or a deer. See if you can identify an animal that feels similar to you, physically. Then take a moment to rest in that experience of your physicality.

In contrast, your mind might feel like another kind of animal altogether. It might feel like a wild horse, eager to run for the sake of running, racing to see what's beyond the horizon, never looking back; unharnessed, unmanageable, untamed. Or maybe more like a turtle: slow and deliberate, a keeper of knowledge, preserving both stories and history for future generations. Or it might seem like a butterfly, a delicate sensibility, flitting from one thing to another. Or a soaring eagle, gifted with enormous vision.

Your spirit might feel like a hummingbird, weighing little, barely physical, easily startled, zooming up into the sky where it feels safe. Or a whale, plumbing the depths, singing strange music few humans hear. Or perhaps you have a coyote spirit, and you often play the role of magician or trickster.

I find it fun to play with this imagery because it can give us insight into our complex nature.

My teachers taught that it was important for humans to recognize our complexity, and to acknowledge that there may be big differences between these parts of us, and to deliberately and consciously work on integrating them. They taught us to seek to understand the particular qualities of our individual Mind, our Body, and our Spirit. It was like sitting down and having a conversation with each our parts. Through that "conversation" we'd come to new realizations about each. Through that process I learned, for example, that I'm primarily kinesthetic. I sense things through my Body first. It's like an intuition, but it doesn't come as a thought; it comes as a physical sensation, a knowing in my body; it's pre-verbal. Those "hits" come to me very strongly, and then I know just what's going on, and I'm prepared to take action.

My Mind is also very strong. I love to learn and I'm very attracted to acquiring new knowledge, especially scientific knowledge. I'm also very skeptical. I don't tend to believe anything unless it also feels true to me in my Body. I can get tripped up, though, when my Body wants to react strongly to something I haven't thought through. Then I need my Mind to step in and cool me down or hold me back. In this way, my Mind and Body work together, as allies.

The third aspect, Spirit, has been a little harder for me to integrate. No doubt this has a lot to do with my religious upbringing. It made me very skeptical of religious ideology, but at the same time I crave a connection with the Divine. I think we all do. The question is: How do you find a safe and stable way to do that? For me, a path opened through connection to Nature. I haven't resolved this question entirely to my satisfaction (as my Mind would say!), but I'm actively working on bringing Spirit more into my life.

In sum, once you get a handle on how each of these different aspects show up for you, you can work on bringing them together in a mutually supportive collaboration. In other words, *we have to work consciously on the integration of Body, Mind, and Spirit*; it usually just doesn't happen by itself. Your Body, Mind and Spirit aren't necessarily working in harmony. In fact, they can each have vastly different agendas at any one moment in time. Imagine! It sounds ridiculous at first, but when you think about it, you can see that it's true. Our bodies, for example, want to be fit and healthy. That's our animal nature. Animals love to revel in their physicality. But our minds can be full of fear: fear of exercise itself, fear of failing to meet some sort of externally-defined image, fear of being evaluated and judged. Out of fear, our mind manufactures all kinds of reasons why we can't do it. We can't make time to do it. We tell ourselves that we want to sit on the couch and watch television instead. And the mind wins, because in Western culture, we think that we *are* our minds, and *only* our minds—when in reality our mind is just one aspect of us, and it's *not* necessarily the part that should be in charge. As a general rule, we don't give our bodies much credit for having intelligence—but they do. Meanwhile, our spirits can pull us out of bodies; we can come to ignore, even denigrate, our physical existence.

So, you can see that these three parts of the human being are very different and often have very different agendas. In addition, our culture and the media in particular seem to exacerbate that sense of fragmentation, pulling our attention this way and that, rarely pausing to explore in depth or help us integrate.

In short, fragmentation and dis-integration are the hallmarks of our age. In fact, we've become so used to it that we think it's our normal state, and most of us don't know there's a better alternative. So when we see someone who has integrated all his or her parts to a high degree, it's startling. Such people embody an astonishing sense of power—*true* power, not just domination or manipulation.

I saw that power in one of my Native teachers, Tu Moonwalker, even though she was gravely ill. She'd had polio as a child and spent many months in an iron lung. But then she recovered—or seemed to. She lived life to the fullest until her early forties when she was diagnosed with post-polio syndrome, a very debilitating disease. People who seemed to recover from polio did so because they grew new nerve connections, but what no one knew at the time was that these new neural pathways were not as robust as the original and therefore not permanent. So, in time, they began to atrophy. And if you had been very active—as she was—they atrophied sooner and more completely. That was her situation. She went from being vital and strong to being wheelchair-bound and, ultimately, oxygen-dependent. But the heroic thing about her is that, by the time she died in 2011, she'd lived twenty years longer than her doctors predicted. In fact, in her final hours she summoned the will and energy to call many of her students, including me, to say good-bye and wish us well. "Don't cry," she said. "I love you. Have a good life." That real-time good-bye was one of the hardest hitting events of my life.[5]

This remarkable woman survived that long because she learned how to command and manage her energy. It was a testament to the power of conscious integration. Once, when I had a private session with her, she reached out and squeezed my hand so hard I gasped. She was so strong in that moment, even though her body was in such a debilitated state. It was because she knew how to harness the power of her body, her mind and her spirit, and how to bring them together. Her power came from the three being equally strong, and nearly fully integrated.

I believe we would all benefit from achieving that level of integration and power. In fact, we *crave* integration and harmony.

And one last point: We must actively create our health and well-being. I once heard someone say, "I may not be working out or eating right, but I'm healthy." I want to challenge that statement, and the assumption that underlies it. Many of us tend to think of health as the absence of disease—but it's much more than that. Health is not the absence of something negative; it's the *active creation* of something positive. If you're not *consciously pursuing your health* by eating right, resting right and working out, you're *unconsciously creating disease*. You're laying the foundation for disease in your cellular structure.

In sum, my Conscious Fitness approach rests on the following principles:

1. Don't listen to your (Scaredy Catt) Mind; Your Mind doesn't always "know" best. Don't let your thoughts hold you back. Listen for the wisdom of your body and your guidance from spirit.
2. A strong Body is the foundation for everything else; it will give you courage.

3. Fitness is a doorway to Spirit; pushing your body's limits leads to greater spiritual awareness. Exercise can be a spiritual practice—it's a way into spiritual practice for those of us who have a hard time starting on that path. Conscious Fitness can help us feel the sacred, while still feeling grounded in our bodies.
4. Body-Mind-Spirit integration is the source of true power. The more integrated we are, the more powerful we are.
5. Your Body, Mind and Spirit don't harmonize without conscious effort; that's why we often feel fragmented, distracted, dis-integrated. My Conscious Fitness approach to exercise—strength training in particular—can help bring about that integration, leading to a surge in positive energy, vitality, and wellbeing.

I want to encourage you to actively create your health and wellbeing by applying my Conscious Fitness approach to your workouts. In this book I'll provide you with the understanding and skills to help you do that. But first, I'd like to share something about how I came to develop my Conscious Fitness approach.

2. My Journey to Conscious Fitness

MY CONSCIOUS FITNESS APPROACH is the culmination of all my years of study, practice, and experience in the world of bodybuilding, fitness, and beyond. Conscious Fitness is more than just theory; I've lived it. It took me to the pinnacle of my sport. In 1986, I won all four of the major amateur titles for female bodybuilding: California State, USA Women's Bodybuilding Championship HW, National Women's Bodybuilding Championship and Ms. Universe. No one had ever done that before.

I was fortunate to be in the sport during bodybuilding's heyday. Truly, it has not been the same since that era and may never be again, a view those of us close to the sport—competitors, photographers and promoters alike—all agree on. It was especially fun to be on the forefront of women's bodybuilding. Back then, we were intent on making it into a serious sport, so we worked very hard and we competed as athletes. Because it was all about muscle and physique, the IFBB ruled out anything that would distract from that. Contestants couldn't wear shiny or sequined outfits; they had to be plainly colored, with no jewelry or props, and our hair had to be pinned up. Now, that's all changed. It's much more about making money, and that means more flash. There are categories called "Bikini" and "Figure," and contestants even wear high heels for those. I'm grateful that I competed when women's bodybuilding was in its purest form.

You might think I achieved this success because I'm special in some way. In our culture, we see a lot of people taking solo credit for their achievements, and we spectators tend toward hero worship. We single out the successful and give them credit that's often beyond what they really deserve. When we do that we diminish our own sense of possibility. We make ourselves small.

The truth is that I am ordinary in many ways. You might say I chose a path, but perhaps it is more accurate to say that a path chose me. I believe that *Conscious Fitness* came to me only because I was willing (and determined) to move through my fears and embark on a process of discovery.

I'd like to share my story with you because I see it as a journey from dis-integration to integration. When it began, I was alienated from my body *and* my spirit, and I relied too much on my mind. In short, I was just like many others in our culture. But I was a seeker, and I was also very curious and open to learning, so I followed my own idiosyncratic path, wherever it led, even to unexpected places.

The Discovery that Changed My Life

I was in my early twenties, and I'd just been laid off from my job at the phone company, so I decided to go down to Mexico for a vacation with some friends from work. While enjoying the beach and the sun, I was also wondering what the future held for me. Little did I know, it was already sneaking up on me.

Body

I was in a little souvenir shop in Ensenada when a handsome blonde guy struck up a conversation with me. We hit it off and he asked for my number. After we returned to the U.S. we carried on a long distance relationship for a time, and then he asked me to move in with him in Northern California. As it happened, he owned a countertop manufacturing shop, and I started working for him in the front office.

Dave liked to run. He was a distance runner, and quite dedicated. He ran three-four times a week, and encouraged me to come along.

The idea of doing something athletic was incredibly intimidating. I'd been craving it for a very long time, but simply had no idea where or how to begin. As a kid, I'd never been allowed to participate in team sports, and I'd been too timid to try anything on my own, so the idea of using my body in that way was a complete mystery to me. Now that someone was encouraging me, I was both scared to death and very open to learning.

I tried running, but I wasn't good at it, and quite honestly, the times I actually enjoyed a run were few and far between. I didn't realize it at the time, but I learned later that I have Thalassemia Minor, a hereditary condition frequent in people of Mediterranean origin. (My heritage is 100% Sicilian.) Because of the condition, my red blood cells are smaller than those of the general population and don't bind iron properly. (Hemoglobin is the protein in red blood cells that carries oxygen. People with Thalassemia make less hemoglobin and have more circulating red blood cells than normal, which results in mild or severe anemia.) Because oxygenation is an issue for me, I'm more capable of activities that involve short spurts of energy rather than the endurance over an extended period that distance running entails. Later, I understood why I was a much better sprinter than I was a distance runner. I didn't know this at the time, however, so I thought it was my failing. Discouraged, I stopped running. Then one day, my boyfriend suggested I try lifting weights.

Dave had built a little workout area in the corner at the back of the shop. I remember there was a homemade plywood bench press covered in green shag carpeting, not upholstered. After work, with regularity, Dave and his two other male employees would go back there, pop a beer, and start lifting.

I was really reluctant to join in. I was embarrassed to try in front of the guys, but Dave kept after me to try it. So I finally did. With Dave's guidance and encouragement, I picked up some weights and tried lifting—tentatively at first. To my absolute astonishment, I fell in love! Instantaneously. Something about that just felt right. And the guys were great. They encouraged me.

I loved the way it felt to push that iron. Immediately, I felt more powerful. The guys got into it; they urged me on and celebrated every time I increased the weight. I had a sense of accomplishment and also progress. I also liked that I was pushing into male territory. No longer was I just a girl standing on the sidelines; I was feeling my own sense of power, and that thrilled me. I loved the whole thing.

After that, I kept coming back for more. I started lifting every day. And I began to feel and see tremendous physical benefits. I saw a change in my body within the first two weeks—and that was wildly empowering for me. Not only was my body changing and improving in really cool ways, but I was also developing a real feeling of strength because I was not collapsing under the weight. For the first time ever I felt that I actually had control over something in my life. *I had control!* You can't imagine what a difference that was for me. You see, I grew up in a fearful household. The reason for this was that my parents were devoted followers of a belief system that instilled fear.

Spirit

My parents were Jehovah's Witnesses. The organization preached that the establishment of God's kingdom over the earth was the only solution for all problems faced by humanity. This would require the destruction of the present world system. Of this, they were certain: it was not a matter of *if*, but *when*. Armageddon was coming—and soon.

The descriptions and graphic images they promoted of what was to come at the end of the world were nothing short of terrifying, especially to a young child. The grown-ups told us kids about fathers watching their daughters being raped. And, in one of the books they gave us to read, *From Paradise Lost to Paradise Regained*,[6] I saw pictures of birds plucking out the eyes of the multitudes of dead bodies lying strewn about the countryside. I was a sensitive kid, and these words and images imprinted themselves upon my psyche.

Growing up in this faith was very difficult for me. I remember some very enjoyable times in the family, but always there was a sense of foreboding, as if a dark cloud hung over everything. It was also a very austere and restrictive way of life. So much so that having fun seemed to be against our religion. We weren't allowed to celebrate birthdays or holidays, for example. Anything and everything outside the faith was considered bad or evil, so I was discouraged from having friends who were not also members of the congregation. I went to a public school, but there was no sense of normalcy there for me. I wasn't permitted to salute the flag or pledge allegiance to the United States of America or even color a picture of a Christmas tree. Because of these restrictions, I didn't get a sense of belonging from school that other kids did. I desperately wanted to be part of things, but I always felt like an outsider.

To me, this was very rigid and isolating way to live. As I've reflected back on it over the years, I've come to believe that my parents did the best they could. They followed the guidelines of their faith, but they weren't nurturing of who I really was. I felt I had to fit into a mold that I just couldn't fit into. And because I couldn't, I experienced a lot of conflict, pressure and stress. I was also expected to be serious about life in a way that a child should not. Because of that early conditioning, I developed the idea that life wasn't happy. It felt like a dark cloud hung over me, a feeling I couldn't shake.

As a kid, I'd loved doing physical things. I was a tomboy, to the great consternation of parents, especially my dad. I was attracted to athletics but, because I was forbidden to participate in team sports, I had no idea if I could be any good at physical things. Later, when I was on my own, I figured it was too late.

Now, suddenly, with weightlifting, a whole new world opened up to me.

I kept lifting whenever I could, and after a while I wanted something more than the workshop could offer, so I joined a little gym. The gym wasn't very elaborate at all; it just had a few weights and not much else, but it was more equipment than I'd ever had access to before and so, to me, it seemed like the world's biggest gym.

By then, I'd gotten very serious about this form of exercise and I started working out there twice a day. In short order, the owners noticed me, and hired me to work in the front office. Not too long after that, I started managing the gym. Something was starting to click; my life path was beginning to fall into place. But there was something missing.

Mind

When I first started bodybuilding, I read voraciously. I poured through all the bodybuilding magazines, like *Muscle* and *Fitness* and *Flex* as well as *Iron Man* and *Muscular Development*, looking to understand my sport more deeply. After a while, however, I came to realize that all the workouts they described were basically the same. They're still selling those same magazines with the same workouts, but there was something missing then and it's still missing now. When the author of an article wrote "Do a bicep curl," for example, it didn't tell me what I was supposed to be *feeling*, what I was supposed to be looking for in my body, when I did that exercise. That was that kind of direction I was wanting, but it wasn't in anything I read.

So I had to find it on my own.

I embarked on what became a very inquisitive, introspective, and interior quest. Because of my upbringing, I had a tendency to question authority; I always wanted to think for myself. So my search was guided by my unanswered questions, and I followed wherever it led.

One of those questions was: *If I want to make this particular muscle bigger, how, exactly, do I do that?* For some reason, I had the intuitive sense that the answer to that question involved more than just the physical realm; I sensed that I had to *think* that muscle into growing, but I didn't know exactly how. So I kept reading, I also did a lot of experimenting. And mostly what I did was *feel.*

Because I sensed that the information I sought could come from almost anywhere, I opened myself up to the possibility of everything I experienced having relevance. Gradually, answers began to come. Without conscious intention, people came into my life serendipitously and gave me nuggets of knowledge I could build on. They included a hypnotherapist, a ballet teacher, and Native American teachers.

All these things conspired, without my directing them, to give birth to a system, which has been further honed over a long period of time by my personal experiences, intuitions and feedback from my clients. Little did I understand at the time that hypnotherapy helped me to command my *mind*, ballet taught me how to work with my *body* in a new way, and the Native teachers enabled me to transcend my fearful resistance and approach the realm of *spirit*.

Body

Meantime, my relationship wasn't going well. I knew it was time for it to end, and I left. Shortly thereafter, another man came along. Bill worked out at the same gym. Before he began dating me he'd dated a woman who was a local competitive bodybuilder, so he knew a little about competitive bodybuilding. He saw something in me, and he began encouraging me to compete. I knew nothing about how to do that, and I was very intimidated—but Bill was very encouraging and supportive. Bill and I are no longer together, but I'm very grateful to him for putting me on this path, encouraging, guiding and supporting me throughout my whole bodybuilding career.

With Bill in my corner, I began training in earnest. I followed a strict exercise schedule and diet. I liked the discipline of this regimen. It gave me a structure for my life and took my mind off my fears.

After about 18 months of hard training, we decided I was ready for my first competitive outing. I entered a competition in Santa Cruz, California in 1984 just to get some stage experience. To me, the show seemed enormous. There were 24 women in my weight class alone.

When you first begin training you're trying to find your way. Everyone's body is unique, so you're trying to discover what *you* need to eat, how *your* body metabolizes. Everyone's giving you advice and you're reading everything you can get your hands on. When I entered that first competition, I was in the lightweight weight class. I was very lean. I weighed just 106 lbs.—too lean, I realized. I'd been on the "lean track," and I'd lost a lot of muscle tissue because I got carried away.

I came in 4th in my division at that competition. I was disappointed, but coming in fourth out of 24 was great in Bill's view.

After the show, Bill gave me some feedback. He said I looked great overall, but that my muscles seemed "flat;" there was no "oomph" to them. So we came up with a strategy to combat that. It involved backing off of carbohydrates for a few days followed by "carb loading" right before the competition. When this technique works, it gives your muscle the look of being shrink-wrapped; you see every vein. When you do things like this, you're essentially making yourself into an experimental laboratory, because it's unpredictable. There's no hard-and-fast rule about how your particular body will respond. I was figuring all this out.

It worked. Then I just began eating more and, going into my second show, the California North Bay, I weighed 112 lbs. This show was smaller; there were just two classes in that show, light and heavy. I was in the lightweight class, and I not only won my division, but I won overall! I beat out the heavyweight champion. I was ecstatic. In just my second show, I'd won!

I admit that, after that, I developed a tiny bit of arrogance. It was good for me, though; it was something I needed to propel me forward. Looking back now, it's almost funny; it was such a small show, but it gave me a sense of accomplishment. And most of all, it gave me the gift of understanding that I didn't need to necessarily "play small" as I'd been taught.

Now that I had a success under my belt, Bill thought it was time for us to make some decisions. He was willing to pay the bills, and so he encouraged me to quit my job and work on bodybuilding full-time.

With that decision, my life changed completely. My days became full with working out, preparing all the right food, tanning, choreography and resting. It may sound crazy, but rest is very necessary because bodybuilding is about tearing down muscle in order to build it up more powerfully. In between, the body needs time to heal and repair. (In general, we grow when we're resting and eating.) Not only that, but posing also requires the expenditure of a great deal of energy. In short, bodybuilder training is ridiculously demanding.

In 1985, after participating in many, many local and regional shows, I entered the California State championship. It was my first statewide show and the biggest there was. I knew it would be tough and I knew that, if I won, they'd be looking for me at Nationals. By then, I'd gone from lightweight to heavy. I competed at 133-135 lbs., so I'd really added weight. Just to put things in perspective, I'm only 5'5" and I was competing in a weight class with women who were 155-160 lbs. and up to six ft. tall.

I took 4th place in the heavyweight class and, while I didn't win, I knew I'd arrived. I got a lot of exposure to photographers and journalists, and buzz began to develop around me. People begin saying that I was the "next bodybuilder on the horizon."

Toward the end of 1985, I entered the National Women's Bodybuilding Competition of the National Physique Committee (NPC), the sanctioning body in the U.S. for amateurs. Now, this was really graduating! The NPC Nationals is a big show with 120 women in the competition. I thought I was ready, but I was also feeling intimidated. All during this time I was reading the trade magazines. In each issue I'd see the big names in female bodybuilding, names like Diana Dennis, Chris Porter, and Susanne McKeon. I realized that I was going to be competing against these women, the best in the country.

For those of you who don't understand the structure of bodybuilding competition, first there's pre-judging, which takes place during the day, and then there's an evening show. Pre-judging is really where all the action is. In the evening, we all participate in a bodybuilding performance, but that is really just a show for the audience. By then, the competition is over and the judges have already made their decisions for the most part.

Pre-judging has three rounds. In four classes, they had to eliminate contestants in order to just get to the top 15 in each. The process certainly weeded out the people who shouldn't be there, but it was harrowing nonetheless because if you didn't make the cut, you were gone. For the first round of pre-judging, they brought us out in groups of five. I remember thinking how all my hard work that year came down to four quarter-turns in front of the judges. *Just four quarter-turns.* Based on that, the judges would make cuts.

I waited nervously for the results—and they called my number! When I learned I had made that first cut, Bill and I were delirious.

Next came the muscularity round. If you're in the first call-out for this round, you know you're doing well because they want to look at the best people first. They began to call the numbers for the first group, and I heard all those big names: Diana Dennis, Chris Porter, and Susanne McKeon. Then . . . they called my number. I literally looked down to check the number on my hip. "*Me?*" I gasped. Everybody laughed.

Stepping back on stage was like a dream. I couldn't believe it. Here I am with all these people, the top stars of my sport! Chris Porter had these amazing legs! But I held my own and, ultimately, I took fourth in that show.

Afterwards Bill gave me some very constructive feedback. He said, when you're up there you look like you're having the time of your life—but you don't look like a winner. There's some other quality you need if you really want to win. Well, I took that as a challenge.

Mind

With Bill's feedback in mind, I talked to a psychologist who practiced hypnotherapy. I asked him if he'd be willing to help me develop more stage presence, to feel like a winner.

Hypnosis is about surfacing issues that lie hidden in the subconscious mind, out of the reach of your conscious mind. Those hidden issues, beliefs, fears—whatever they are—have tremendous power; they limit us in ways we don't understand, let alone consciously agree to. Hypnosis is about finding those obstacles, those things hidden in your subconscious that are stopping you, and releasing whatever's there so it no longer gets in your way.

The truth is, I'm a big skeptic. I love science; I love the process of investigation and discovery—and I love that science requires testing to prove that something works. In addition, my experience with the cult pretty much inoculated me against taking things "on faith," or believing things just because everybody else does. Ask all my friends! I question EVERYTHING. I like to think for myself. So, even though I'd initiated the idea of hypnotherapy, I was suspicious of it working.

In our sessions, the hypnotherapist worked on my feeling "lesser than," my not feeling like a winner. I remember a specific post-hypnotic suggestion he gave me one day: "You'll go out today feeling lighter and brighter." When I went back outside, I could see a brightness I'd never seen before. The landscape seemed to go on forever and everything was very sparkly, almost like there were diamonds on things. I started to think this might work.

His other post-hypnotic suggestion was that, the next time I stepped on stage, I would feel like a winner.

My next show was my return to the 1986 NPC California state competition. I remember being in the "pump room" backstage where all the bodybuilders prep for the competition. You oil yourself up and maybe you do some work with weights there because you want to get your muscles big and engorged with blood right before you go on. In the background, you've got expediters organizing all the contestants. In other words, it's chaos, and your brain is on overload.

When the expeditor called my group we all got in line, and I felt the same as always—excited, nervous and uncertain. But then, the second I put my foot on stage, a rush of energy washed over me. What was that? I asked myself. Then I remembered: *I am a winner.*

This was the major turning point in my career. That year, I became the first to win all four of the major women's bodybuilding titles.

After I won the Nationals in 1986, things took off. Joe Weider—"the" big name in the sport of bodybuilding—took a liking to me. He upgraded my flights, so I flew first class to Singapore for the Universe contest. When I won that, they sent my picture over the AP wire back home so my friends would know I had won. That next year, 1987, I got to travel the world. I'd written to the IFBB and offered to do guest appearances for free so long as the promoter who hired me covered business class or better airfare and expenses. They agreed to let the promoters of the worldwide federation know, and so I went to Belgium three times, as well as Malaysia, Grenada, and Trinidad and Tobago to name a few. In between, I also did World Mixed Pairs show with J.J. Marsh in Madrid and the World Pros show in Nice/Cannes.

I was having a blast, just a great time. Everything was great except that I also had to do the Olympia, the top professional show,

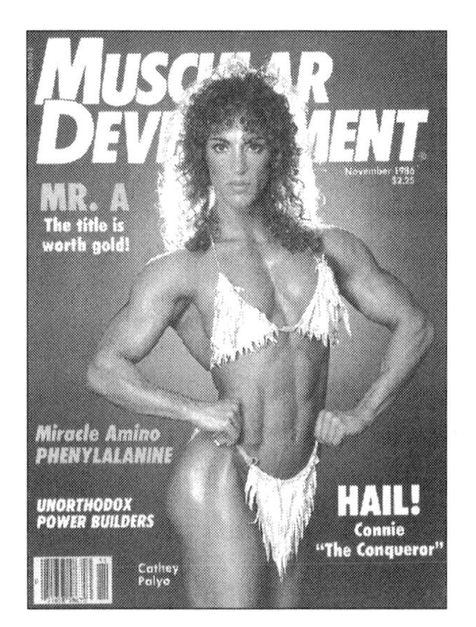

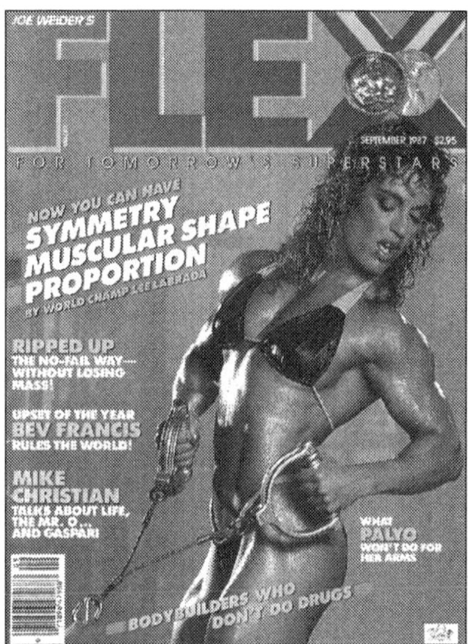

that year. But, all the traveling was too disruptive. It was impossible to maintain a steady regimen, and so my body was just not where it needed to be. I came into the contest heavier than I would have liked, and I placed poorly.

After that, I rested a lot. Then I began to prepare seriously for the Ms. International competition, a very prestigious professional show put on by Arnold Shwarzenegger, now known as the Arnold Classic. I worked very hard to prepare, and as a result, I had a completely different body—I was in my best shape ever. I won the Ms. International title in 1988.

I competed in one more Olympia and then Dave Zelon's USA vs. USSR in Moscow in 1989. I retired shortly thereafter. My success in bodybuilding opened the doors to the gym business, which is where I am today.

What are the Lessons from My Story?

Bodybuilding shaped me in countless ways. Bodybuilding taught me that I'm stronger than I think I am.

Bodybuilding made me stronger in my *body* despite all the doubts in my mind. It helped me to see that the limits I had put on myself and my dreams were not real: they were like a box I drew around myself to keep myself safe and small. I drew those limits because of the fear that was always there, the fear that was instilled during my childhood. I had all kinds of fear: Fear of not being good enough, fear of failure, fear of standing out, fear of going after what I wanted. It took a long time for me to get the courage up to try new things until one day I realized I was bumping up against the same thing every single time: *my own sense of limitatio*n. And then I began to see that this is a made-up thing. It was just a product of my *mind*.

This was the first inkling I had that my mind wasn't necessarily my best ally. I figured if I was going to do anything at all, I had to trick myself into it: I had to learn how to bypass my mind. So I adopted a kind of code: *Go do it. Act on what you want; don't let your thoughts hold you back.* None of this came naturally; I always had to "push my personal envelope." I didn't think of myself as being athletic, but I found I could *build my body anyway*. I was afraid of competition—after all, I'd never really had any experience competing with others for anything—but I could *compete with myself* and, in that way, I found I could win competitions.

I learned that if I stretched beyond those imagined boundaries, nothing bad ever really happened as I may have imagined it—even though my mind literally *screamed* at me that it would! But it didn't. In fact, whenever I pushed past those boundaries I always ended up getting something out of it, and I always had a good time! This served me in competitions and in my life afterwards. The first sport I tried after bodybuilding was rollerblading. It was petrifying at first. I was afraid I'd fall or hurt myself in some way, or even worse—that I'd hurt my ego! But I pushed through that fear and got really good at it. Then I started mountain biking. And pretty soon we were doing that five or six times a week. Then I moved on to snowboarding, then yoga and now, most recently, to golf. The first time I walked into a yoga class, for example, I was terrified because my mind was saying, "What are you doing? You won't be any good at this! You don't take classes—you learn on your own." But then I stopped those thoughts from taking over. "The people in the class weren't good at it either when they first started," I said to myself. "You have the right to be a beginner. You just go out and learn." And then, when I went on to start and run my own business—you can't imagine the terror that brought, and continues to bring! But I keep moving through it, because if you *don't* try, your likelihood of failure is 100%, whereas if you go ahead and try you've at least raised your odds to 50-50!

By working through my body, I learned to discipline my mind. By strengthening my body, I learned how to transcend my mental fears. I could have given in to those fears, let them define my life, but something told me not to. Even now, I ask myself how I got myself out of that situation: raised in a cult that diminished its members and discouraged personal ambition. Bill used to say that something deep in my being told me that if I didn't push back, I wouldn't ever get out; there was no graceful exit. That something was *spirit*.

I knew that, to survive, I had to be strong. But I didn't really believe I was strong because I was so full of fear. Something—my spirit—told me that if I made my body strong, it would help me succeed despite all my doubts. Spirit was right. Having a strong body has served me at every turn. Bodybuilding kept me strong for the other things I wanted to do later in life, post competition, and it forced me to be gregarious and open. Because of bodybuilding I learned to develop an alternative persona. I was fearful inside, but I could appear to be fearless on the outside. Bodybuilding also got me through car accidents, and snowboard and mountain bike falls. Would I have held up that well if I hadn't done all that lifting? No.

Contrary to popular opinion, bodybuilding is not just about lifting weights, as in: "I pick them up, I put them down." Bodybuilding is an art, and your muscles are your media. And like all arts, it has transformative potential. There's an element of the ancient shamanic practice of shapeshifting in bodybuilding. One of the things that first captivated me about this sport was that I saw changes in my body in just a few weeks—and then I began to notice that changes were occurring not only in physical body, but also in the way I looked at the world. Some of my limiting beliefs began to fall away. I was experiencing some of the magical power of shapeshifting.

In this book I'll share with you how my Conscious Fitness approach can be applied to strength training in order to help you integrate mind-body-spirit to maximize your workout. But first, as preparation, I'd like to share with you some more perspectives about each of aspects of the essential triangle of Conscious Fitness: Body, Mind, and Spirit.

3. Body

AN INTIMATE JOURNEY

I WANT YOU TO FALL IN LOVE a little. With the human body. With *your* human body.

As much as we walk around in our bodies, we're not very intimate with them. They're the *miracle we take for granted*.

So first, I'm going to review some incredible facts about the human body, and contrast that with the state of many of our bodies today. Then, I'm going to take you on a tour of some basic anatomy so you get a sense of how your body works from a muscular perspective.

And finally, I'm going to ask you to take all that knowledge and turn it into admiration, gratitude—and then love. Because if you truly see all the things your body does for you, how amazing and marvelous and functional it is, you will fall in love with it. Because despite whatever superficial imperfections you may focus on, your body serves you well. It does myriad things for you every day. And if you love your body, truly love it, you will want to nurture and support it by eating right, keeping it fit, and taking care of it through rest and relaxation. And never, ever take it for granted.

That's our goal for this chapter. So let's begin.

Your (Amazing) Body: A Primer

I want to share some incredible facts about the human body—your body:

- Three times per minute, your blood circulates through your body. It travels 12,000 miles/day—the equivalent of four cross-country trips. In fact, laid end-to-end, you have 60,000 miles of blood vessels in your body, more than twice the distance around the earth.
- Your heart pumps 2,000 gallons of blood every day.[7]
- The amount of electricity a full-grown human brain generates is enough to run every telephone in the world–all at the same time with enough left over to power even more.
- Every inch of your skin has 32 million bacteria on it; the vast majority of those bacteria are not only harmless, but also necessary for your survival.
- Nerve impulses from the brain travel up to 170 mph.[8]
- Our eyes receive approximately 90 percent of all our information, making us basically visual creatures.[9]
- The average human heart beats 100,000 times a day, 40,000,000 times per year—and about 3 billion times in a lifetime.[10]
- When you gain a pound of fat, your body makes seven new miles of blood vessels. Your heart must work harder to pump blood through all of these extra new vessels, which may put a strain on it, and reduce oxygenation and nutrient replenishment in other tissues. Fortunately, if you lose a pound, your body will break down and re-absorb those now unnecessary vessels.
- Pound for pound, your body produces more energy than the sun.
- We will take about 600 million breaths in our lifetime.[11]
- Approximate number of body cells in the average human: 100 trillion.

- Every cell contains estimated 6-8 feet of DNA.
- We are about 70% water.
- We breathe 23,000 times/day.[12]

No End in Sight: The Illusion of Limitation

I always had this sense that our bodies could do much more than we thought. I was fascinated by stories of mothers being able to lift a car if their child were trapped underneath. While it might be that adrenalin was partially responsible, the fact was that the body could do it. The question for me became, how could we tap that potential? Could we learn to do that at will?

In Michael Murphy's groundbreaking book, *The Future of the Body: Explorations into the Further Evolution of Human Nature,*[13] he makes the case that the human body is still evolving. He calls our attention to 12 attributes of the body, citing these as evidence of enormous, yet-to-be-fully developed potential. Perception is one of those attributes. There are extraordinary examples of perception being extended in all kinds of ways. Some wine tasters, for example, can make ten thousand discriminations, and there are perfume testers who can make 30,000 distinctions. People can train their eyesight to far greater acuity than was ever thought possible. There is growing evidence of extra-sensory perception, as well. People can be trained to perform remote viewing, as they did at the Stanford Research Institute.

Another attribute Murphy cites is our ability to love. We can expand our capacity to love through the practice of love. Our relation to pain and pleasure can also be developed. We can learn to induce states of pleasure, and there is evidence that we can learn to control pain. This had a huge impact on me.

If you look around today you can see copious evidence that we are still evolving. The slogan of the 2008 Olympics was *Higher, stronger, faster.* And, in fact, the Olympic athletes who competed in China did perform higher, stronger and faster. They broke more than 40 world records and over 130 Olympic records. Where does it stop?

Some species can even regenerate missing limbs. Science is working on understanding how that's possible so that, someday, it may even be possible for humans to do the same. There are many new human capacities being developed all the time. An article in *The American Psychologist* (August 1994) entitled "Expert Performance" reviewed dozens of studies about abilities that were thought to be genetically determined, such as perfect pitch or the ability to remember strings of numbers on a single hearing or various athletic skills.[14] These studies have shown that everybody who is trained can learn perfect pitch, can learn to extend their short-term memory, and can extend their athletic abilities. It was a landmark study, one of those great historic roundups of the evidence.

There's more evidence, too. In just a few years we learned how to navigate with cars—several thousand pounds of steel streaming down a highway at 60-70, even 85 miles per hour, making lane changes, stopping and going, only a few feet from each other. This is not an ability we had 100 years ago. Back then, we would not have had the ability to navigate all that complexity. But today we can. Some kids' kinesthetic sense is amazing, giving rise to extreme forms of sports, like skateboarding or Parkour. Other kids seem to have been born with a "mouse" in their hand.[15] In 2009, Juan Enriquez gave a TED talk about the evidence for rapid evolution. *Will our kids be a different species?,* he asked.[16] We just don't know where the body can go.

Those are just physical abilities. There are also emotional capacities, cognitive skills, and spiritual abilities. Every single human attribute gives rise to the extraordinary — among men and women, young and old, in all cultures.

We develop all these new abilities without even realizing it. So why would we voluntarily put limits on ourselves?[17]

The Future of the Body was a tremendous catalyst to my bodybuilding investigation. I kept asking myself, how could I push my body in ways that would make that evolutionary leap? How could I push it into places that people hadn't gone before, specific to my sport? I took these questions very seriously, and I sensed the answer lay in the mind-body connection: Could I push my muscle to grow by making a deep connection with it and actually *commanding* it to grow? That was always the game. More than winning on stage, it was mastery over myself that I was after. Of course I wanted to win, but winning was never my prime motivator. It was to be the best that I could be. If someone was better, so be it. If they beat me, they were better. But for me to get mastery over myself, over how I looked up there on stage, that was the game. I wanted to be in the most peak condition I could possibly be in.

So that's what's possible: incredible potential. But where are we now? Where are *you* now with respect to your body? Let's look at some statistics.

The State of Our Bodies Today

- Only half (48.4%) of adults 18 years and over met the 2008 federal physical activity guidelines for aerobic activity.
- Just over 1/5th of us (22%) still smoke.[18]
- Over a third of Americans (35.9%) 20 years and over are obese. Childhood obesity has more than tripled in the past 30 years. In 2008, more than one third of children and adolescents were overweight or obese. Even more concerning, we now we have an epidemic of overweight infants. Productivity loss due to obesity will cost the U.S. economy more than $580 billion per year by 2030, unless something changes.
- An estimated 1 in 10 Americans report depression.
- One in every three children born in 2000 will develop Type II diabetes in their lifetime.[19]

- According to former U.S. Surgeon General, Dr. C. Everett Koop, of the 2.4 million deaths that occur in the United States each year, 75% are the result of **avoidable** nutritional factor diseases. That number is said to be conservative.
- Today, for a thirty-year-old person, the odds are **95 out of 100** that he or she will suffer and die from a degenerative, nutritional factor disease (such as Cancer, Heart disease, Stroke, Diabetes, Alzheimer's, Parkinson's arthritis, etc.).[20]
- 2011, 16.7 million Americans (6.5 percent of the population) were dependent on alcohol or had problems related to their use of alcohol (abuse).
- In 2010, approximately 7.0 million persons were current users of psychotherapeutic drugs taken non-medically (2.7 percent of the U.S. population)[21]
- Abuse of tobacco, alcohol, and illicit drugs is costly to our Nation, exacting over $600 billion annually in costs related to crime, lost work productivity and healthcare.[22]

I think these statistics begin to paint a picture of a nation **out of touch with our bodies**—and increasingly becoming more so. I want to change that. This chapter is a start.

Creating an intimate relationship with your body

Visualization is so important, because once you begin to "see" your body, you're on your way to creating an intimate relationship with it. You can begin to converse with your body. I mean this both figuratively and literally. "Converse" means to *turn with*.

We must learn to move *with* our bodies, meaning move in ways that are in tune with our body's nature. Our body can teach us how to do this, if we attend to it. Each body part—each muscle—has its own personality; there are things that are easy for it, and things that are not. If we listen to our body and feel into our muscles, they will tell us what we need to know to support them.

Your Muscular Structure: A Guided Tour

In the gym, I often take people to anatomy chart so they can see what's under their skin. If you look at how the body is put together, you see an almost mechanical thing: a system of cables and pulleys and, in a simplistic sense, that's what it is. Most of our joints work like levers, though some (like the patella or kneecap) work like pulleys.

Here are some examples of the mechanical feel of a lever-type action.

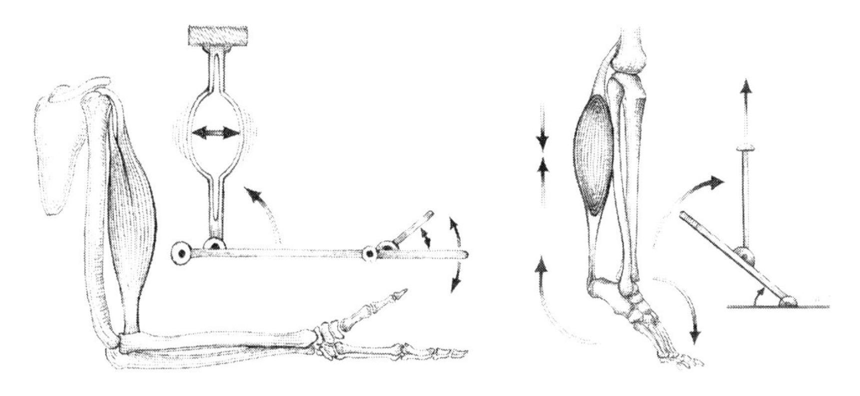

As you look, you begin to see how each of your muscles works and how they work with each other. You see how your muscles are attached to your bones by tendons, and your bones are attached to each other with ligaments.

It's not essential to understand this in great detail, but a general understanding is important because it helps you to develop a felt sense of your body. When you understand the basic structure of your body, you begin to develop a feeling for how your bones, muscles, joints and tendons and ligaments work together. This helps you understand how best to work your muscles, and also how to avoid injury.

Many injuries arise because we don't understand how our bodies work. We do exercises incorrectly, putting undue strain on our joints or tendons, which are actually quite delicate. Exercise involves putting stress on various parts of our bodies in order to build muscle; we need to understand where to put that stress such that we accomplish our goals without injuring ourselves. It takes a while to develop this "body wisdom," but the ability to visualize how our body is constructed is key. That's why, in this section, I'm going to take you on a guided tour of the major muscle groups so that you can get familiar with your body.

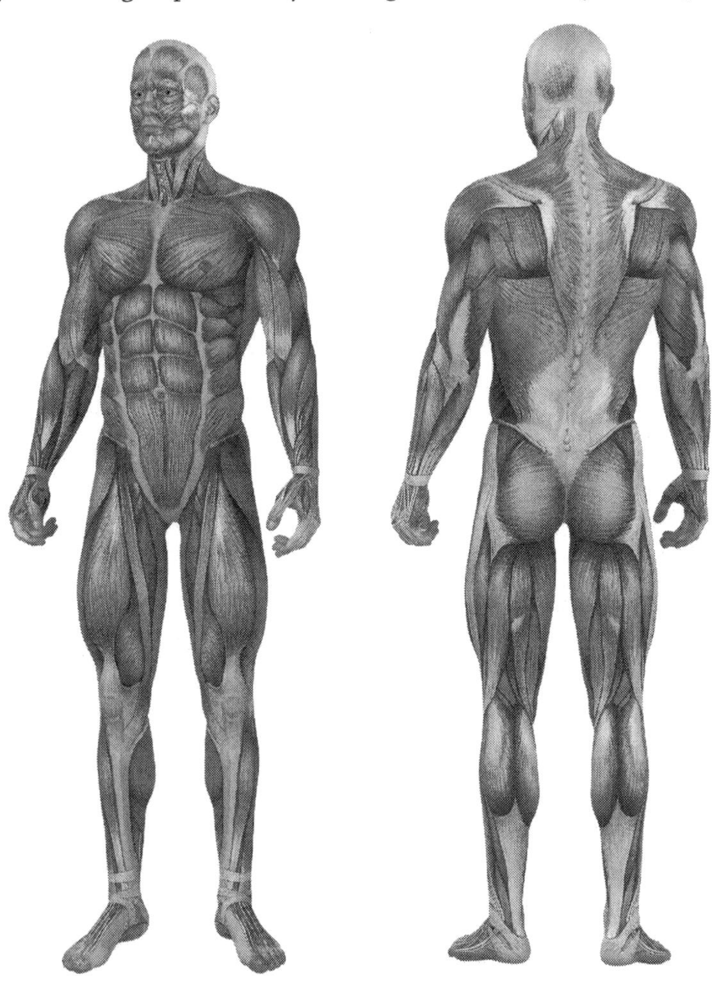

Getting to Know Your Upper Body

Let's start with the muscle located in your upper back area and around your neck.

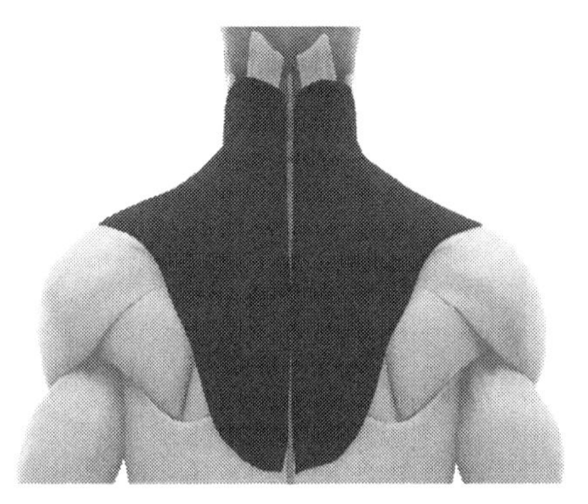

That's the **trapezius** muscle. It's called that because, as you can see, it's shaped like a trapezoid. The trapezius muscle is responsible for the movement of your shoulder blade and neck. It also assists with breathing.

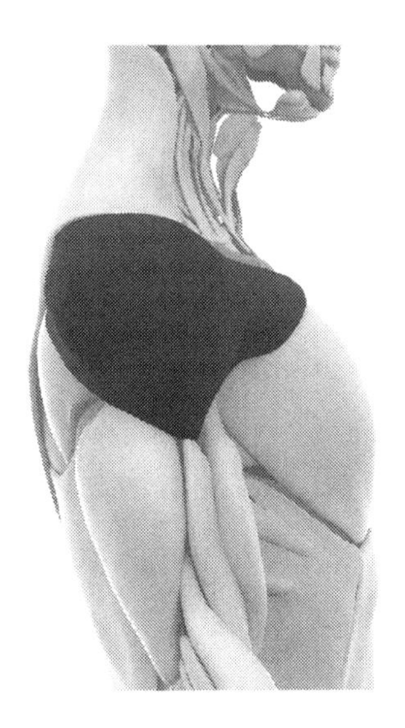

Next to the trapezius muscle is your **deltoid**: your shoulder muscle. Your deltoids are responsible for moving your arms forward, backward, and to the side. When you lift something overhead, you're primarily using your deltoids.

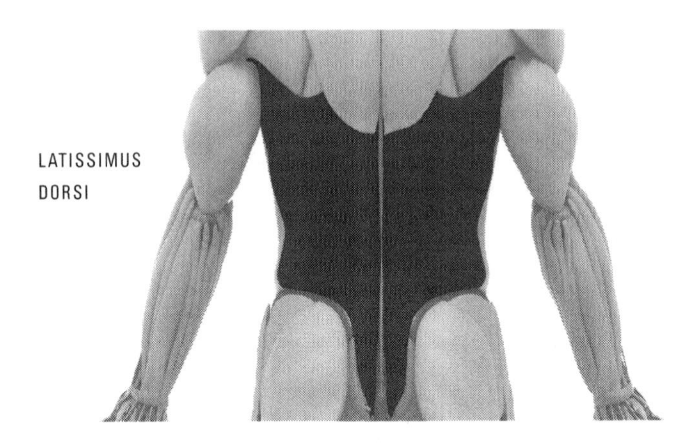

The back consists of the **latissimus dorsi** (or "lats"), **rhomboids and teres.** The lats are the larger muscles of the back. Your lats enable you to extend your arms and rotate them medially. They're also responsible for a pulling action. For example, when you bend over and something pull toward you, you're using your lats. When well defined, the lats look like wings.

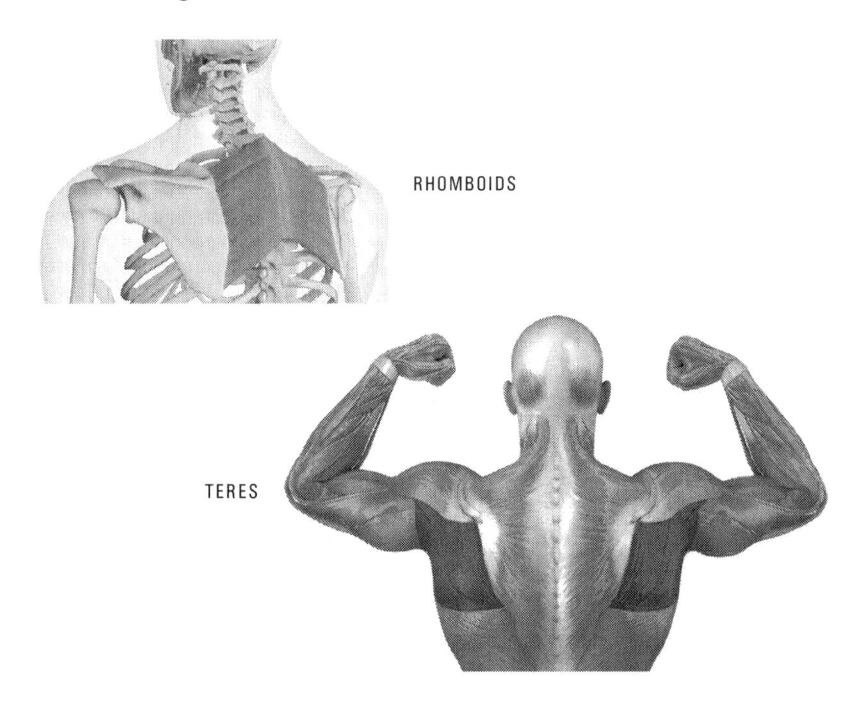

Your **pectorals major, or "pecs,"** are located in the upper chest. Your pecs enable you to flex and adduct the arms, enabling you to bring your arms toward the center of your chest.

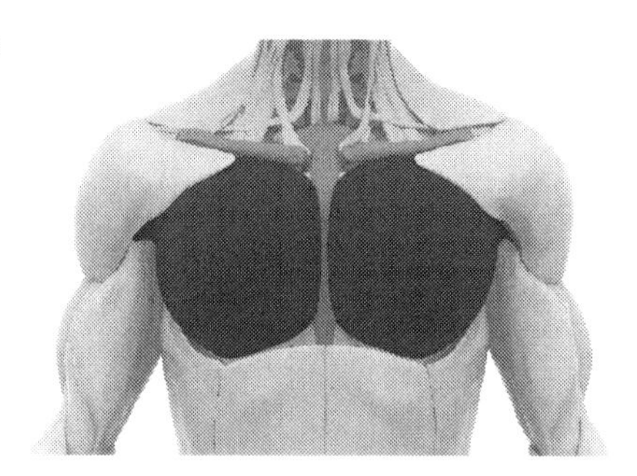

Another important muscle is located within your upper arm, the **biceps brachii** (or just biceps). Your biceps control the flexion of your arm, enabling you to bring your forearm in closer to your upper arm as when you do a bicep curl.

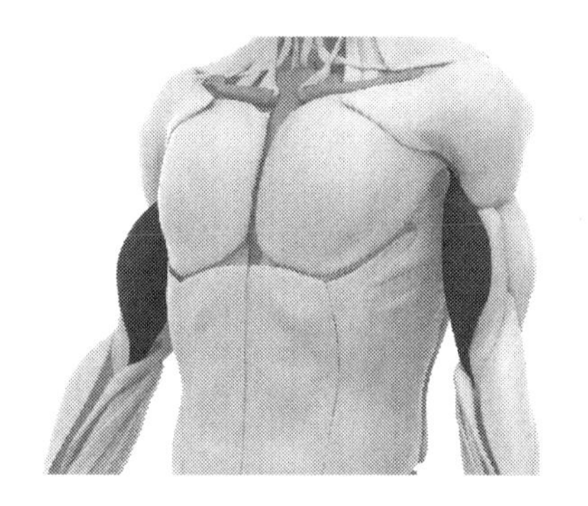

The counterpart to the biceps is the **triceps brachii** (or just "triceps"). It's located on the back of the upper arm. The triceps brachii enables you to extend or straighten your arm.

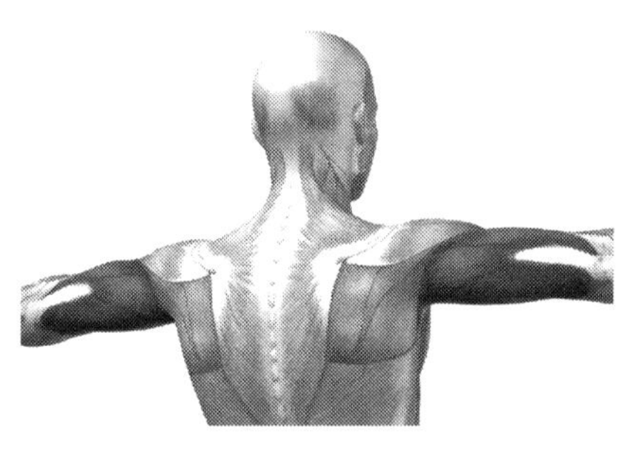

On the front of the torso are your **abdominal** muscles. These enable you to flex and rotate your spine, enabling you to bend sideways.

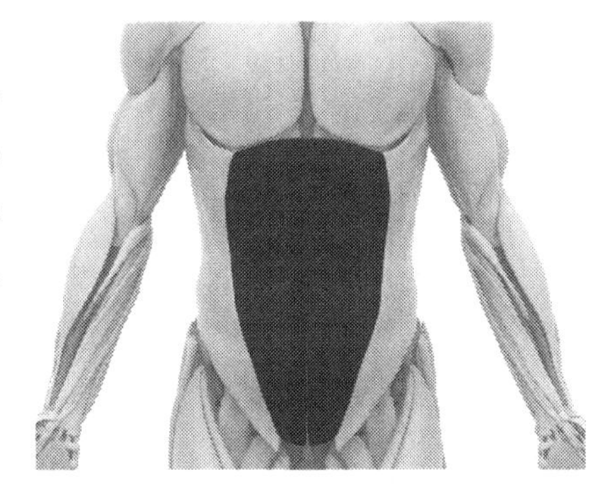

Your Lower Body

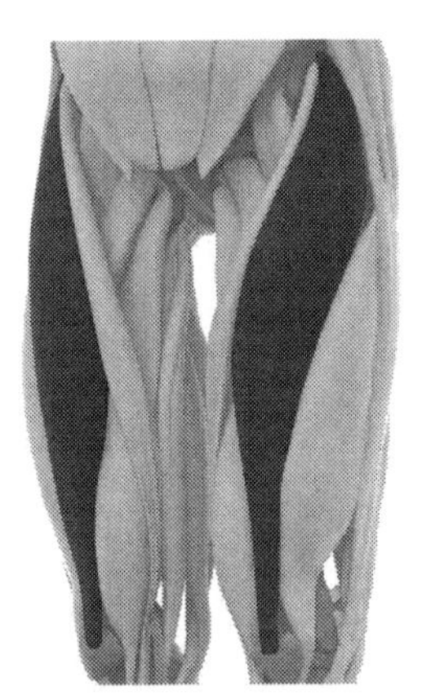

The **quadriceps** is a group of four muscles located on the front of your thighs. The quadriceps muscles help you to *extend* your knee.

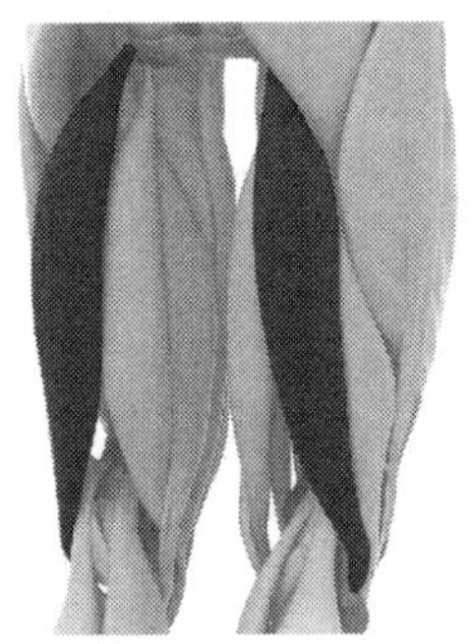

The **hamstrings** are the muscles located on the back of the thighs. The hamstrings enable you to *bend* your knee.

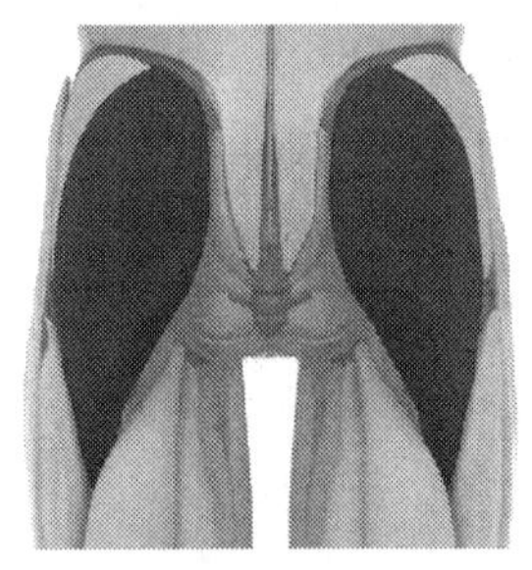

The **gluteal muscles** (glutes, for short) are a group of muscles responsible for *hip extension* (moving your leg backward from your hip) and *hip abduction* (enabling you to move your leg away from the midline of your body).

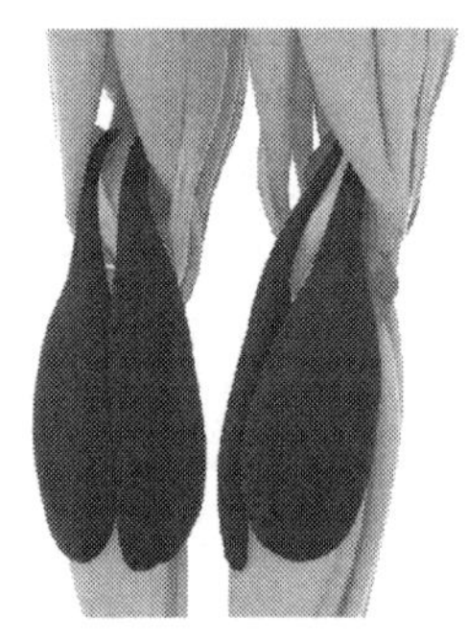

The **gastrocnemius**,—also known as the calf muscle—is located at the back of your lower leg. Together with the soleus muscle, it helps you to push off for walking and to stand on your toes.

The Relationship between Muscles, Ligaments and Tendons

Our muscles hold us up and hold us together. They do it through tension. You know those little plastic toys where, when you push a button, the whole thing collapses? Think of your skeleton that way. It would just collapse down onto the floor like those toys if it weren't for the dynamic tension of your muscles.

The muscle-skeletal system is a *tensegrity* of muscle and bone, meaning the muscle provides continuous *pull*, the bones discontinuous *push*. The forces between the bones and muscles are held in balance. This forms the basis for all of our physical mobility. Muscles are what cause the bones to move. People tend to think the joint is doing the movement. No! The joint is just a well-oiled hinge. All the power comes from the muscles.[23] Muscles also act as support for the joints.

Ligaments

The ligaments' job is to attach one bone to another; in brief, they hold your skeleton together. Ligaments help stabilize the joints and provide

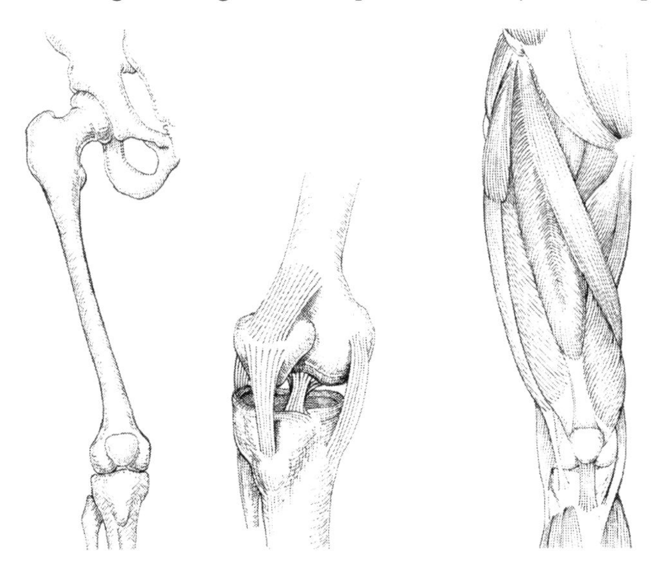

a structure for the bones. To help you understand what I mean, let's take a look at your knee.

The ligaments on the knee criss-cross in order to hold your knee in place and prevent your femur and tibia bones from moving backward or forward. Ligament tears usually come from a violent movement, such as turning your ankle.

Tendons

Tendons are the bands of connective tissue at the end of your muscles that attach your muscles to the bone, thus enabling your muscles to pull your bone. Notice how the big, thick muscle of the quadriceps gets narrower as it becomes a tendon. It goes from thick, meaty and red to white, narrow and delicate.

Why is it important to understand something about ligaments and tendons? When you work with weights, especially, you want to make sure that you're using your muscle to lift the weight, not a ligament or tendon, because these can tear if you put too much of a strain them. You also want to make sure you're using the *strongest* part of the muscle, and that you're not moving in a way that puts undue stress on a ligament or tendon.

Strengthening the ligaments and tendons that support your muscles can help you further develop your muscles.[24] This is all the more reason to not put undue stress and strain on them. Don't work the tendon, but work the muscle and it will communicate with the tendon.

Making an Intimate Connection with your Body

It's not essential to understand any of this in great detail. There's no reason to memorize the names of the various muscles. What's most important is to "see" them, and to begin to understand how they work to move our bodies. When you understand the basic structure of your body, you begin to develop a felt sense of how your bones, muscles, joints and tendons and ligaments work together. You begin to develop a visual and felt sense of how best to work your muscles. That general, "felt" understanding is important for one critical reason: it helps prevent injury.

You want to understand the relative *strength* of each major muscle so you don't overtax it, or ask more of it than it was designed to give. Many injuries occur because we put undue strain on shoulder and knees joints. The muscles in these joints are actually quite delicate and intricately configured. If you visualize those joints in your mind's eye before a lift, you will have a much better sense of what you are asking of that muscle.

You also want to know how the muscle you want to work is configured. You want to know where the meatiest part is and also where it tapers into a tendon that attaches to the bone. You need this understanding because, in any given exercise, *you want the tension to be on the thick, meaty parts of your muscle(s)* and *not* on your tendons, joints, or ligaments, as that's a recipe for injury and a less effective workout.

It takes a while to develop this "body wisdom," but visualization is key. *Use visualization to become intimate with your body – how it's put together and how the parts work together.*

Visualization is so important, because once you begin to "see" your body, you're on your way to creating an intimate relationship with it. Then you can begin to converse with your body. I mean this both figuratively and literally. As I said before "converse" means to *turn with*. It bears repeating that we must learn to move *with* our bodies, meaning move in ways that are in tune with our body's nature. Our body can teach us how to do this, if we attend to it. Each body part—each muscle—has its own personality; there are things that are easy for it, and things that are not. If we listen to our body and feel into our muscles, they will tell us what we need to know to support them.

When I think about what my Native teacher accomplished with her body, overriding that debilitating disease for so many years, I know there is no limit to what we can accomplish when our bodies, minds and spirits are aligned. It's been proven over and over that we can create new neurological pathways. And once you begin to make that intimate connection with your body, you just keep learning; it doesn't stop. I've been practicing yoga for 11 years, and I'm still blown away by the fact that I can still I feel something I've never felt before; I can still accomplish something I couldn't before.

4. The Gym Within

GETTING YOUR MIND IN SHAPE

BECAUSE OF THE WAY I had been conditioned by my upbringing, I experienced a lot of fear. It was almost suffocating. I was afraid of trying new things, especially in groups. I longed to be athletic, but participating in sports in school was forbidden. Because I'd never played a team sport, I had no confidence in my abilities, which led to more fear. Because I had no experience, I didn't know if I was any good, I was scared to try. I was afraid I'd fail other people, or embarrass myself.

It wasn't until I tried weight lifting that I began to sense that I might be good at something physical. It was positively thrilling.

The Jehovah's Witnesses discouraged independent thinking and always told us what to think, but I tended to be very inquisitive by nature—persistent in my wanting to understand. I was also a very introspective kid, perhaps because I couldn't understand the world I was told to believe in.

These qualities came into play as I began to practice weightlifting more seriously. I became quite curious about my own process. For example, I began to notice how often my thoughts were doubtful or fearful. I'd set goals for myself, but then the conversation in my head would tell me I couldn't possibly do that number of reps of a certain exercise, or that I couldn't possibly lift the weight I had in mind. I began to observe myself, as if from a distance. I noticed that, if I listened to that voice, I'd stop myself, but if I put those thoughts aside and just concentrated on *doing* it, I could accomplish what I set out to do—and far more.

I started realizing that my *mind* was a real problem. It got in the way of the sheer physiology of what I was doing. I became very aware of how I could let fear limit me. Then I thought back to the stories you'd hear about women—mothers—who can lift a car if they need to free their child trapped underneath. To me that meant that, physiologically, we have the innate ability to do that, but it's blocked in some way; we just can't seem to access it unless we find ourselves in extraordinary circumstances. Why not? And what if we could? How might we learn to tap into that hidden potential? How could I control my mind so that it wouldn't get in the way of my making things happen? These became my driving questions.

These early explorations set me on a path of learning how to manage my mind; how to move it aside when it was obstructing me—and how to use it to achieve a desired effect.

This path to empowerment started with one simple, yet profound realization: my thoughts aren't synonymous with *me*. My thoughts are just my thoughts—and I could decide whether to act on them or not.

With that fundamental realization, I could step back and notice my thoughts in a kind of dispassionate way. I could be curious about them. How was my mind going to react to this particular situation? What was it going to try to get me to do—or, more frequently, *not* do? And why?

Bodybuilders always diet before a competition, and I remembered overhearing some talk about how they felt about dieting. They would often express how tired they felt. Soon I realized that they'd been told by other bodybuilders that dieting was extremely difficult, and that their workouts would be harder, so they started saying it, too. But by saying those things out loud, they were actually setting themselves up. They were conditioning themselves to expect that they'd be weaker with less body weight, and it became a self-fulfilling prophecy. Instead, they could be saying more empowering things to themselves, such as: I'm getting leaner, stronger, and my energy level is much greater than before.

As I practiced becoming the witness to my thoughts, it began to feel like the person telling me to doubt wasn't *me*, but a separate self—one that I didn't have to listen to. I didn't have to always take my thoughts seriously. This gave me tremendous freedom to invent my responses. In particular, it gave me a way of approaching the resistances to exercise and fitness that my mind often presented.

Hypno-Fitness: Harnessing the Power of the Mind

Previously, I recounted how hypnosis helped me learn how to act like—and be— a winner. Many years later, I became a certified clinical hypnotherapist. To my great astonishment, the formal training confirmed many of the things I had already been doing, naturally and intuitively. Here's what I discovered.

As I've said, my mind was often filled with fears. Perhaps my successful experience with hypnosis early on in my career planted a seed. In any event, I began to see how these fears didn't serve me. Then I began to notice how, in order to keep me from doing things, my mind would even tell me things that weren't true! It would tell me to put limits on myself—even when the limits weren't real and didn't need to be there.

Once I understood that, I was determined to find a way out. I began to think that, if I could quiet my mind, that would release more of my potential. So I experimented with that, and it worked! When I quieted my mind first, I could lift more.

To quiet my mind I had to detach from all the "noise" inside. With that detachment came a new level of appreciation: I began to see that my mind was like an instrument, an instrument of light and energy.

Yes, it could be chaotic and diffuse, running all over the place. Yes, it could put up all kinds of obstacles and barriers to stop me and keep me safe in the status quo—but I could also take control of it and use it as a tool. I could *concentrate its power* and *focus it with intention.*

When I applied this *focused concentration* to weightlifting, it began to transform in pretty magical ways. At the time, I didn't understand exactly why. But then, when I began to study for my certification as a hypnotherapist, it was like all the lights came on. I began to understand the theory underlying what I had already been doing intuitively in the gym. This gave birth to the technique I use in Conscious Fitness that I call "hypno-fitness." Here's how and why it works:

Hypnosis may seem a bit mysterious to people, but it's quite simple, really. In essence, it's a technique that helps *quiet your conscious mind while also bringing your body into a profound state of relaxation.* When that happens, the doorway to the subconscious opens.

Our conscious mind tends to hold onto a lot of limiting beliefs and patterns. It is our conscious mind that tends to hold us back. Out of fear, it can tell us that our body isn't capable of doing things that it actually *is* capable of doing. When it does this, our mind essentially *separates* from our body. This diminishes our spirit and ultimately makes us more fearful, weaker, less integrated and less powerful.

Our subconscious, however, is a field of unlimited potential.

Hypnosis opens the doorway to our subconscious while also helping our conscious mind to release those old stories of restriction and limitation. When you free yourself from these, you can do things you never thought you could. That's because our mind, body and spirit are no longer working at cross-purposes; they're working together. One captivating example is the story of the runner, Lee Evans. His coach used hypnosis to help Evans train. On the night before he was to run a major race, he rehearsed every single stride of that race, over and over, under hypnosis. As a consequence, when he went out to run, *his mind and body were one.* Evans took the world record in the 400-meter dash in 1968.

You, too, want your mind, body and spirit to work together. That's the key to reaching your potential, and it's the central idea underlying this book. Later, we'll speak more specifically about my hypno-fitness technique applies to lifting. Right now, I want to focus on *your* mind in more general terms by speaking about how to get it in shape so that it supports you in becoming the best you can be. In this chapter I'm going to do three things:

1. Give you some key information that will inspire, excite and motivate you to get to the gym—or, if you've let your motivation lapse—get *back* to the gym.
2. Explain why you have to "fire your mind" when it comes to exercise—because your mind just isn't going to be on your side, so it shouldn't be in charge.
3. Give you some tips for how to manage your mind so that it doesn't get in the way of your getting fit, but actually helps you do so.

So, let's get started.

The Mental Benefits of Exercise

There is a scientifically proven way to make yourself smarter: Go for a walk or a swim. Yep, it's a fact. Neuroscientists and physiologists have been gathering evidence of the beneficial relationship between exercise and brainpower for more than ten years, relating exercise to everything from improving learning in kids to staving off dementia in older adults. But they didn't know exactly *why*. Now some new findings are making it clear that mind-body "isn't just *a* relationship; it is *the* relationship."

Exercise appears to build a brain that resists physical shrinkage while enhancing cognitive flexibility. Exercise, the latest neuroscience suggests, *does more to bolster thinking than thinking does.*

A study in the *Journal of Applied Physiology* said that the key may lie in the effect exercise has on our mitochondria, the tiny structures inside cells that supply the body with energy. Exercise stimulates the body to create *more* mitochondria: "Just as a booming metropolis might build new power plants to meet a rising need for electricity, *our muscles respond to the demands of exercise by producing new mitochondria.*" It appears that the brain "adapts and changes by bringing more of these powerhouses online," J. Mark Davis, a physiologist at the University of South Carolina, says. The increased energy supply allows the brain to work faster and more efficiently.[25]

To my mind the word "demand" stands out. *Demand* means pushing yourself. Demanding more of yourself is what stimulates the creation of something new. As bodybuilders, our goal is to build muscle. To do that, we have to demand more of our muscles, so that the body has to creatively adapt. If you don't push yourself, if you keep going to the same place every time, your musculature is not going to be forced to change. But if you *do* push yourself, you get even more benefit. Moderate exercise stimulates your DNA, and vigorous exercise changes it even more.[26]

Assuming this finding about mitochondria is true, exercise can help us "power up" our brain, leading to improvements in listening skills, cognitive skills, everything. That is very cool. Expending energy actually leads to the *creation of* new energy sources.

There are implications for aging as well. We naturally lose mitochondria as we age, but exercise may reverse that. "The evidence is accumulating rapidly that exercise keeps the brain younger," says Davis.

It's Not What You Think: The Workout Paradox

Remember the last time you engaged in strenuous physical activity? If you do, I bet you remember you felt great—you felt a good sense of tired. You probably ate well and slept like a baby.

It's the same with a good workout. You feel great afterwards: strong, and powerful and tired in a really satisfying way. But then what happens the next day? You forget how great you felt, and you don't want to go to the gym. So you make up excuses. I call this the "workout paradox," and it's the number one problem we face. Exercise feels so good, and yet we don't want to do it. We love the effect it has on us, but every single time we resist doing what will get us into that wonderful state again.

I know, because it happens to me, too. *Right*, you say, *I don't believe you. You live to be in a gym.* No. It's a problem for me, too. It's a problem because, frequently, our minds are not supporting our bodies. Our bodies know what's good for us, but our minds aren't tuned in.

So I can say it definitively: *exercise is energizing.* How many people really get that? This is one of the things I talk about to people in the gym almost daily. I'll spot someone I haven't seen for a while, and I'll ask, "Where have you been?" Inevitably, they'll respond by saying something like, "Oh, you know my job...I'm so tired when I'm done. I just don't want to come in." And I tell them "Come in, you'll actually leave with more energy."

This is a huge part of the workout paradox. We tend to think that exercise is only an *expenditure of energy* when, in reality, it's a *source of energy*. That may seem counter-intuitive, but it's the truth. Study after study has proven it: exercising will actually give you more energy.[27]

How Does Exercise Increase Energy?

Regular physical activity can improve your muscle strength and boost your endurance. Exercise and physical activity deliver oxygen and nutrients to your tissues and help your cardiovascular system work more efficiently. In a vigorous workout, your heartbeat increases. As your heart beats faster, it pumps more blood, which then surges through the brain. Your brain cells absorb more oxygen, and you feel more mentally alert and energetic. And when your heart and lungs work more efficiently, you have more energy to go about your daily chores.

Better-conditioned muscles also make daily tasks that much easier. When you exercise, your ability to recruit and use muscle fibers are increased so you require less effort to perform any physical task. And as you become stronger through exercise, so does your immune system. Being sick drains us of energy. Exercise boosts immunity, and strong immune system helps avert illness, or at least reduces its length and intensity.[28]

Tim Puetz of the University of Georgia notes that their analysis found that nearly every group studied – from healthy adults to cancer patients to those with chronic conditions such as diabetes and heart disease – benefited from exercise. He acknowledges that it may seem *counterintuitive* that expending energy through exercise would increase feelings of energy and reduce fatigue, but he points out that previous studies have shown marked increases in the levels of energy-promoting and mood-enhancing neurotransmitters such as dopamine, norepinephrine and serotonin in the brains of animals that are placed in regular exercise conditions.[29]

More about the Mind-Body Connection

Working out helps everything. It's a balancer. It's a regulator. It's been proven that it helps relieve stress and anxiety.[30]

But here's something that blew even my mind: Is it possible that *just thinking about exercise starts the process?* Yes, it is. In a fascinating experiment, researchers at the Cleveland Clinic Foundation discovered that you could *strengthen a muscle just by thinking about exercising it.* A group of thirty young people performed imaginary exercises by focusing on the muscle in either their little finger or their elbow. At the end of 12 weeks, those who focused on their pinky improved its strength by 35%, and those who focused on their elbow, by 14%! There was no similar improvement in the control group, which didn't do this mental exercise.[31]

What are the implications? For one, it reinforces the idea that there *is* a connection, that **our body and our mind are intimately connected**; they are not separate, as we have been taught for so long. We are made up of disparate parts, but these parts are all intimately interconnected and in communion with one another.

Our thoughts can affect our physical wellbeing. Correction: Our thoughts *do* affect our physical wellbeing—and vice versa. So if we can manage our minds and *direct* our thoughts, we can positively affect our bodies. Therefore, when you're in the gym, turn off the TV and put down that magazine! Otherwise, your body and mind are not connected. How can you think about what you're doing if you're distracted? If music is blasting in your ear, how can you "hear" the vibration of your body? How can you feel it? How can mind and body communicate with each other if you're actively trying to distract your mind? Keep your body and your mind connected and engaged with each other. The benefits are far-reaching.

Getting your Mind in Shape

I want to talk now about a few things you can do to help get your mind on your side. Remember, *you're in charge*, **not your mind!**

Resign from Resignation

Often, when I hear people speaking about their lives, I hear a kind of resignation in their voices. "This is just how I am," they'll say, or "I'm just how my mother was." Yes, you may be of a certain height or tend toward a certain body type because of your inherited characteristics, but there are still many things you can change for the better. The power is within you. We see this in the research being done on gene expression now. We used to think that just HAVING a particular gene meant we were predisposed—even destined—to have a certain disease. But that is not necessarily so. Genes can be turned on or off depending upon certain circumstances in our lives. Environmental factors such as where we live, what we eat, who we interact with, when we sleep, how we exercise and aging can, over time, cause chemical modifications around the genes that will turn those genes on or off. New information surfacing about the brain indicates that it is far less fixed and far more adaptable than previously thought. The neuroplasticity of the brain means it has the potential to reorganize itself by forming new neural connections to adapt to losses caused by injury or disease.

In sum, very little is set in stone. You have a lot of control over your body, your health and your life. So don't give up before you even begin! Don't resign yourself to being less than you can be. I know from personal experience that the body is very pliable, very plastic. There are many possible shape changes. So don't limit yourself prematurely. Instead, focus on possibility and keep testing yourself to discover what your body and mind can do when they work together.

Here's an example. A 62-year-old man at my gym had been working out for 20 years before I met him. He told me that he had a frozen shoulder and back problems. When I spoke to him about these things, he just shrugged. He thought his days of improvement were over. He was afraid to work the muscles of his core because of back issues. He was so fearful about his workout that he always did it in a very controlled way—so it never changed. He had resigned himself to the same workout all the time, with the same results. The way he motivated himself was through his journal; he kept careful records of every workout—which is quite a wonderful technique.

When he said "I know how to keep my back from getting hurt," I felt how resigned he was to the status quo; he expected that his back would be a problem forever. I sensed that wasn't necessarily so; I sensed he could actually go much farther than he thought. But rather than trying to take him there right away, I started slow. I asked if I could work with him just a little, and he agreed. So I started showing him how to do one new thing at a time, and then layering one new thing upon another. Bit-by-bit, he changed; his back got stronger. As his back got stronger, he became stronger all over. Now, he has muscles on his legs he never had before. He can do 12 pushups and all kinds of other things he never thought he could. "I was so sore for four days," he said, "But now I feel great! I never, ever thought that I could do this. It's amazing!"

How you view your body, your *beliefs* about it, are very important. Don't focus on your perceived limitations; focus on possibility. Start to test your body to see what it can do, to see if it can move beyond the limitations you've put on it with your mind. Be willing to explore, to be curious, and pleasantly surprised. I think of this as "callous-ing" your mind, making it a little tougher a bit at a time, so it doesn't shut down and stop you.

I had, long ago, a friend who was a paraplegic. I remember seeing him at the gym where he'd strap himself onto the bench to do dumbbell presses or use a raised bar on a Smith machine to do pull-ups out of his chair. This is how he forced himself to continue moving. He kept at it, and he saw real gains, and he started to feel differently about himself. It freed him up so much that he started singing opera. You see, it's about always pushing that envelope—that envelope where we keep our limiting beliefs and expectations about what's possible. It's about testing those assumptions, always in a conscious and safe way.

Avoid Negative Self-Talk

We all need to take personal responsibility for our lives, for making them as good as they can be. It starts there. Sure, there may be things you can't change—but how do you know until you try? As we've talked about previously, human beings are constantly acquiring new abilities. It's part of the evolutionary process. That's the cool thing for me: We don't know where this goes. What portion of our brains do we really use? 1/10th? What other latent capacities do we have?

But often the stories that we end up telling ourselves limit our capacities.

Not verbalizing limitations is important, in my view. This is especially true with respect to aging. Today there are anti-aging supplements and drugs and modalities (strength training, yoga, etc.) out there. So why stop just because you're 60 or 65 or 75? Where is it written? I say if I want to mountain bike at 75, and I feel capable, then that's what I'm going to do. There's no law that says I shouldn't.

I say, *be limitless*—at least *don't tell yourself a story that limits you before you even try*. If you bump into a limitation, then work with it. But don't build limits in ahead of time.

Set Realistic Goals

Being in the gym business, I see many people set themselves up for failure. I see people who, when they first join the gym are very excited, very committed at that moment, and so they go overboard. They'll say their goal is to work out six days/week. They probably think that'll please me. They're surprised when I say to them, "Let's get more realistic and make this something you can handle, consistently."

This tendency to over-commit is the other side of the "limitation coin." In the heat of the moment, we forget that we do have complicated lives with multiple responsibilities.

This happens because of what I call the "all or nothing illusion." It's a product of the extremism we see in our culture. We think we need to go all out, but going from guardrail to guardrail with no moderation in between actually sets us up for failure. We tend to over-commit and then, when we find we can't keep the commitment, we quit altogether.

So, in the end, we get nowhere. It's like we think of ourselves as an "on-off" switch. Well, that kind of thinking isn't sensible and it's not going to help you get fit.

Fitness is not about overdoing. It's about *doing*. Period.

Competitive bodybuilding is a good example of what I'm talking about. It's extreme, admittedly. It asks people to do extreme things with their bodies in terms of both exercise and diet, and there's something very addictive about that. As a result, many people got caught up in that addiction. But even when I was involved in bodybuilding, I found a way to do it sensibly. If I was able to stay balanced in such an extreme environment, you can too. You just have to become aware of the lure of the "all or nothing illusion"—and sidestep it.

In my view, the first step in any fitness program is to set a realistic intention. Ask yourself: *What's my desired level of fitness, based on all the parameters of my life?* Take some time with this question. Get real.

I say "get real" because we are susceptible to imagery planted in our consciousness by the media. But the images people see in magazines—particularly those like *Muscle* and *Fitness* or *Shape* or *Men's Fitness* or *Flex*—are ideals that are not attainable by most people leading normal lives. One of my least favorite things about these magazines is that they have an investment in turning elite athletes into mythic, otherworldly superheroes. This is especially appealing to teenage boys.

These magazines create these myths by writing things about these athletes that just aren't true, printing digitally enhanced photos, and not revealing that many take massive amounts of drugs to help them attain their physical appearance. It's sensationalism. Basically, these magazines are catalogues for products. These aren't real stories; they're lead-ins for ads. It's all very subtle, but very manipulative. I know from firsthand experience.

These magazines participate in perpetuating the all or nothing illusion because they reinforce the idea that the goal is some kind of physical perfection. This has a sapping effect on our motivation. *If we can't be like that,* we think, *then why try at all?* And people give up—or they live vicariously through the fad diets and workouts the magazines promote.

I'm here to say you don't need to do that. Fitness has nothing to do with how you look. **It's about you having control over your body and your life**. Today, very few of us feel that sense of control—for a variety of reasons. Exercise—fitness—can give it back to you. Being fit is not that hard or unattainable, and it's a logical way to live. So, free yourself of all that outside-imposed imagery, and *imagine yourself fit, vibrant and healthy.* Embed that vision in your consciousness by picturing it every day. It's *you* you're focusing on, not some image in a magazine.

Then, based on your specific intention, set a goal that feels do-able, achievable, that fits into your lifestyle—a goal that stretches you a bit, but doesn't overload you. Ultimately, everyone's goal should be to *move every day*, somehow, and move with weights at least twice every week. But if you're just beginning (or beginning again), the goal you're looking to set is whatever you feel confident about doing *consistently*. Don't over-commit to exercising six days/week at the very beginning. That'll just set you up to fail.

If you set a modest, moderate goal of say, moving with weights two or (if it feels do-able), three times/week, you'll have a better likelihood of success. Remember, even if it's only two times/week, you're already *33% better* than you were before! You'll feel good about yourself, which is very, very important. You can build on that.

A Word about Consistency

I believe consistency is one of the most important aspects of fitness. It's about turning fitness into a habit, making it into daily practice. That daily practice may simply mean you take the stairs instead of the escalator or you park your car further away from your destination or you take your dog on a longer walk on those days that you're not in the gym. Developing consistency is about finding those things that will help you stick with your discipline, with getting your body moving. When you show up consistently at a gym, you get to know the place and the people better. Consistency breeds consistency.

Consistency is about realizing that every workout doesn't have to be epic; it doesn't need to be the biggest, baddest, hardest workout ever. Yes, there are real benefits to pushing through barriers—but we don't have to do that all the time. For the layperson whose goal is staying fit and healthy, you don't need an hour-and-a-half in the gym every time. It would be great to have a good, solid hour at least 3 days/ week. Then, if you don't feel like it the other days, come in and just do a half-hour of cardio. Because consistency is more important than the amount of time you spend. And *inconsistency* is the surest route to falling off the wagon, permanently

So, the bad news is there's no quick fix. There's no miracle, no magic bullet. There's no piece of equipment, no pill, no technology that will do it for you; you can't "shake weight" your way to health and fitness. You can't melt all the fat off your abs in just five minutes a day, no matter what the ads say. The only thing that creates fitness is moving your body on a regular basis: getting up off the couch and moving.

The good news is that getting fit is really much simpler than you think. It just takes a commitment to work out consistently. And there's more good news: What you'll find is that *your system actually craves discipline*. As a culture we've pursued leisure and comfort to the extreme; we've fooled ourselves into believing that's what our bodies want. But that's a fiction. In actuality, our bodies *want to be used*. They hunger after it. So there's a huge reward awaiting you.

5. The Spirit of Conscious Fitness

Keeping your Body Healthy is an Expression of Gratitude to the Whole Cosmos - the Trees, the Clouds, Everything.

–Thich Nhat Hahn

Touching Peace: Practicing the Art of Mindful Living

THERE IS A SPIRITUAL DIMENSION to health and wellbeing—and fitness.

Our culture is very materially oriented. We have been taught that the material and non-material realms are very different, governed by very different laws and principles, and so we have a difficult time integrating the two. As a consequence, many of us operate from a very deep split at the core of our being; we are either predominantly spiritual or predominantly material in our way of being. Few of us are in balance. Yet, these are both equally important aspects of the larger Whole, which is All One.

My Native teachers made a key observation about modern life in our materialistic society: the more we break away from spirit—true spirit, not illusory dogma—the more sickness we experience. The farther we get from this essential connection, the more pathology we create: not just physical sickness, but all kinds of sickness. The rise in addictions in our society is, I believe, symptomatic of that pathology. Addictions are symptoms of misguided attempts to get to the other side, to find that connection, to get into place of total relaxation and integration—but drugs and alcohol fail you in the end. They're just impersonating the real thing all the while luring you into a dependency upon them. Why not seek integration in a way that honors and benefits the body, making it stronger?

Another aspect of that spiritual malaise is that many people in our society feel isolated and alone. I know that when I feel down, that's where my mind goes. It feels like I'm the only one having these feelings, that I'm the only one who can't take a day off, can't get organized, can't get what I want. Almost everyone seems to have had this experience, but we feel all alone anyway—and now it seems that feeling is becoming a worldwide plague. Figures released by the Council for Evidence-Based Psychiatry in 2014 would seem to bear that out. Their report states that sales of antidepressants have skyrocketed everywhere in the industrialized world. More than 53 million prescriptions for antidepressants were issued in 2013 in England alone. This is almost the equivalent of one for every man, woman and child, and constitutes a 92% increase since 2003. In Denmark, if the prescriptions were equally distributed, every citizen could be in treatment for six years of their life.[32] The situation is even worse in the U.S. because of the direct advertising of prescription drugs to the public.

That sense of isolation may be one of the drivers of the over-consumption that characterizes our society. We want what we imagine everybody else has or is, and if we can't have that, we need to indulge ourselves in some other way.

The truth is, however, that we are anything but isolated and alone.

Science is now telling us what indigenous spiritual traditions have always taught: that the nature of the Universe is relationships. Here's how Paul Hawken stated it:

> *The first living cell came into being nearly 40 million centuries ago, and its direct descendants are in all of our bloodstreams. Literally you are breathing molecules this very second that were inhaled by Moses, Mother Teresa, and Bono. We are vastly interconnected. Our fates are inseparable. We are here because the dream of every cell is to become two cells. And dreams come true. In each of you are one quadrillion cells, 90 percent of which are not human cells. Your body is a community,*

> *and without those other microorganisms you would perish in hours. Each human cell has 400 billion molecules conducting millions of processes between trillions of atoms. The total cellular activity in one human body is staggering: one septillion actions at any one moment, a one with twenty-four zeros after it. In a millisecond, our body has undergone ten times more processes than there are stars in the universe, which is exactly what Charles Darwin foretold when he said science would discover that each living creature was a 'little universe, formed of a host of self-propagating organisms, inconceivably minute and as numerous as the stars of heaven.'*[33]

Recently, I came upon a *Scientific American* article that talked about how human beings are in collaboration with the bacteria that live in our bodies.[34] The article was eye opening because of what it revealed about our nature: the human being is not one solitary, separate being, but a kind of "group project." It reminded me of something my Native teachers taught, which is that we humans are made up of all these different components: organs, blood, muscles, bones, stem cells, platelets hormonal glands, emotions. We're a walking collaboration of all these disparate parts. It's really quite miraculous that all these different aspects are able to coordinate with each other to keep us functioning—and yet we take this all for granted. Not only that, but here we are trying to kill off bacteria all the time. With all the focus on anti-bacterial soaps, hand sanitizers and antibiotics, etc., we're doing this on a grand scale. We're bent on destroying the very things that are helping us!

My point is that we've been largely unconscious of how much support we have from the rest of creation. When we're successful, we tend to think we did it all alone—which feeds our ego, but also our sense of isolation. And when we feel like we're failing we think that we're all alone and helpless. Neither is true. We're surrounded by support. The rest of creation gives this support to us ongoingly, unselfishly, and we're indebted to it for our existence; we're deeply dependent upon the sun, the air we breathe, the microbes that improve the soil that grows the plants and nurtures the animals that become our food. We're especially indebted to water, which comprises 60% of our bodies (and even a larger percentage—75%—when we are infants).

This "extreme interdependence" is not a matter of faith or belief; the scientific evidence supports it.

I think that realization shifts things profoundly. I think it means we need to exhibit more awareness of how connected we really are to the web of life. I think that should give us a real sense of power—not the kind of power that arises from ego, but the power that arises from knowing we are a part of something larger than ourselves and that we are co-creating the future of our planet together with all the other beings that are here with us on the planet at this time. With that awareness comes a profound sense of gratitude—and also responsibility.

Out of that awareness arises **a commitment to become the best you can be**. It's a commitment to your own healthy functioning for the benefit of all.

I think people give up when they think their lives don't matter. But what if that's not true? What if everyone matters because our lives are not just ours? What if our lives are meant to serve a larger purpose? I *believe I have an obligation to make myself better so that I can contribute to the evolution of the species and everything going forward.* Maybe I'm not going to be the next Nelson Mandela or Mother Theresa, but if I can positively influence five people today, and they can positively influence five people in their lives . . . the world gets a little better. I believe we all have that obligation to try to contribute, in whatever way we can, each and every day.

That's how fitness became for me a spiritual practice.

I'm human, and so I forget this connection all the time. That's another thing my Native teachers taught: human beings are forgetful.

We forget our sacred relationships; we forget that we are part of One Whole. We forget that we are gifted every day by the abundance and generosity of Nature all around us. So we need to remind ourselves to feel grateful for all the support we've received. I think we would all benefit by paying more attention to our good fortune. We need to anchor ourselves there, in gratitude for all we've been given—even the hard things—and for life itself. If we anchor ourselves there, and if we forgive ourselves for being human, it makes it easier to be scrupulous with ourselves, with how we lead our lives. If we have compassion for ourselves, that helps us look more critically at what we fill our lives with—is it mindless television, mindless eating, pleasure for its own sake? Are we binging on food or abusing alcohol or drugs? If so, we must ask ourselves what purpose do these things serve? Are we acting in ways that are worthy of all the gifts we've been given?

The Body-Spirit Connection

All the great spiritual traditions talk about the care of the body. They all see it as important. In fact, in the early beginnings of Western medicine, concerns of the body and spirit were intertwined. But with the coming of the scientific revolution and the enlightenment, these considerations were removed from the medical system. Today, however, a growing number of studies reveal that spirituality may play a bigger role in the healing process than the medical community previously thought.[35]

I believe that working our physical body feeds our spirit.

For one thing, it makes us feel accomplished. It's that feeling of putting in a hard day's work, or that you've really done something. I think that sets up for the rest of our day or evening or following day. I think it makes us better for all our relationships, whether those relationships are with our kids, husband, wife, friends, boss, co-workers, customers or pets. These relationships are all better for that expenditure of energy.

If you reflect upon everything that goes on in a typical day, all the information and energy we take in, you can begin to see how taking some time to let that out, to *expend energy* is a great thing. It's like the breathing out. Yes, we expend energy during the day to accomplish various things, but I believe that expending energy by exercising is very different from expending energy doing things like reacting to problems or daily demands, which can drain you. Exercising replenishes you because it's energy spent *for you*. That's very different from expending energy to make a living.

Exercise can help us de-clutter from the day, so we can shed the layers of static that have attached themselves to us. That's another aspect of the benefits of working out: after exercising, we think with a clearer mind.

As we've discussed, expending energy through exercise actually brings you more energy, but only if you do it joyfully, not as a chore. When you surrender into it, you receive back. This is another way in which exercising becomes spiritual practice. You experience a different type of tiredness after a workout: a good and peaceful tiredness.

Lifting also gives me this incredible sense of appreciation for my own body, for the way it functions and serves me every day while asking so little in return. It's pretty awesome, and fills me with gratitude.

I want this for everyone. I want people to experience this sense of communion. Because otherwise we're walking around in these bodies, but we have no idea how remarkable they are. We're born into our bodies, and we just tend to take them for granted; we don't take the time to build a relationship with them. If you don't spend time in communion with your physical being you're prone to one of two illusions. One is the illusion that your body is outside your control, which makes you feel powerless. The other is that is that your body is completely yours to control.

Neither of these is true. As that article about the bacteria reminds us, our bodies are a team effort—and we need to learn to be a good member of that team.

Can Fitness Help Evolve our Consciousness?

The great spiritual teacher Aurobindo once wrote, "the better organized the form, the more capable it is of housing...more developed consciousness."[36] To me, that expresses perfectly why fitness is also a spiritual practice. A body that isn't sufficiently exercised tends toward entropy. It's frankly amazing how quickly muscles atrophy. That's why, when you're hospitalized for any reason, the attendants tend to get you up and walking as soon as possible. It's because remaining in bed, just like remaining sedentary, leads to the fast breakdown of muscle. And this, of course, plays into a descending spiral: we feel weak, so we don't exercise, which makes us weaker.

As our body's vibration drops, our physical form becomes disorganized and out of harmony with our other aspects; this leads to disorganized thinking and a dampened spirit. It downgrades our consciousness, especially when we couple it with poor nutrition. When we're in that state, we're vulnerable to being preyed upon by the negative aspects of our culture: distracting, meaningless television and movies; entertainment disguised as news that tells us what to think, but not why; advertisements that encourage us to ask our doctors about pharmaceutical prescriptions, but not about how we can prevent illness, not about how we can improve our overall health and wellbeing.

Aurobindo knew this. He knew that a fit, organized body was the best home for our spirit.

When you practice physical fitness, you're organizing your physical form and increasing its capacity for achieving even higher states of consciousness. And, just as your muscles weaken quickly, they also respond very rapidly to increased use. After all, that's what they're *for*. Have you ever needed a service and wandered into an establishment where at first you found the workers on duty just sitting around bored, but then they seemed leap to life because now they have a job to do? Well, those workers are like your muscles. They're longing to be called to action.

Many people think they can become spiritually attuned without attending to their bodies, but I'm not sure that's really possible.

Our bodies are the base foundation for everything else. That's why it's important to ensure that our bodies are vibrating as strongly as they can. Your body houses your mind and connects you to spirit. If your body's vibration is choppy or out of balance your mind feels this, and it won't work well. If, however, your body is healthy, it will help your whole being to come into harmonic resonance.

That's why I'm so concerned with the epidemic of obesity among our nation's children. If you have to use your creative mind to lift yourself out of your circumstances, how creative are you going to be if your mind is dulled or slowed by a non-vital heaviness in your body? Underprivileged kids, especially if they're obese, are particularly vulnerable to this dis-integration. That's because, the heavier our physical form gets, the more we risk losing the connection to the higher vibrations. If we could help obese kids learn to move, to attune their bodies, would that help them to pull themselves out of poverty? It's empowering to be fit and healthy.

Look at what people in the past have done to awaken their spirits. The ascetics, for example, engaged in self-flagellation and extreme fasting. Other spiritual seekers sit in meditation for days on end or participate in vision quests, etc. These spiritual endeavors are actually all about the body. It's all about clearing a space for spirit, isn't it? It's about pushing the body to such a limit that finally it opens. Your physical being goes away and it opens to the next thing. *Pushing the body to its limits leads to a greater spiritual awareness.* Just think about how you feel when you've had a really good workout. You feel extraordinarily alive! And in good cheer, because you feel *integrated.* That's the key. Exercise, fitness, and eating right—all these things can help you with that integration process. They help you feel more whole.

Spiritual teacher Andrew Cohen talks a great deal about the importance of consciously creating the future—not just letting it happen to us, but actively creating it. To do that, he says, you need to *free yourself.* "Free yourself from mental slavery," sang the late, great, reggae artist Bob Marley. For me, that begins with the physical. It's a logical, grounding place to start. It's easier to start there because we can feel it when we transcend it; we can feel the liberation.

So I believe we can achieve more in the spiritual realm by beginning with the body, as it's the base foundation of our being. That's why lifting weights can be a spiritual practice. How do we transcend gravity and go into outer space? We use booster rockets. Weights are like personal booster rockets. By lifting weights you can transcend the physical. When you lift you push out of this plane and break the barrier between you and something greater. Lifting weights teaches us to push into new territory, into possibility. *Lifting weights can lift our spirits.*

Spiritual Benefits of Conscious Fitness

One time, when I returned home after having been gone for many years, I found myself taking my Mom to task for not preparing me for life: "You were so ready for the world to end that you didn't teach me how to live, how to make a living!" I cried. Her reply was, "You should've been happy just cleaning toilets." I'll never forget her saying that. It's not that I wouldn't clean toilets for a living if I had to, but I wanted more. And I wanted it to be OK that I wanted more.

As time went by, I kept asking myself, why did my mother believe that? The conclusion I came to was that the Jehovah's Witnesses strongly reinforced the idea that you should not stand out. Everything associated with the JWs was drab, and your pursuits were supposed to be humble. Your main goal in life was to spread "the Word." That was the prime directive; nothing else was important. It was a very non-egoic teaching. This message of non-striving got through to me at a very young age, before I was able to think on my own, and I still contend with it today. I struggle with thinking that I shouldn't be creating my life and that I don't deserve the success I've obtained. I struggle with this inner voice whenever I feel the urge to do or create more.

But the urge to create is also very strong in me, as I believe it is in most people. I don't believe this desire comes from ego.

My Native teachers taught that the Universe is *creative*. It creates every day, whether new cloud formations, rainbows, sunsets, or new life forms. Nature creates for its own sake, because that is its essence. Indigenous people honored the creativity they saw all around them through their art. When they made art, they felt they were participating in that universal flow of creation. Through their art making they became one with that universal creative force.

I feel something similar when I lift weights. I've found that the discipline of physical exercise on a regular basis puts me in a special place: it puts me in tune with my body. When I lift, I feel a sense of communion with myself, with my true self. I have insights I wouldn't ordinarily have. It's given me a deep intuitive sense about the body, how it works and what's good for it.

When I'm in this state, I'm slowed down and I'm really focused. I can feel my breath come in and I can decide where to direct it. I choose a specific muscle I want to oxygenate—the muscle I'm working on in that moment—and I can see oxygen being transported there. In those moments, I'm using breath as energy.

From this place, lifting weights feels like painting a wall, brushstroke after brushstroke. It feels consistent, smooth, seamless and rhythmic. It's about finding the right vibration, being in a flow of energy that's beyond us, as in the practices of chi gong or tai chi. I often experience synesthesia, so when I reach that state I can actually hear the muscle humming: a beautiful, rich, satisfying hum. This is how I believe many artists must perceive reality. Their perception is so keen, so elevated, that it links them with the spiritual realm.

As a consequence, I can "read" other people's bodies and know instinctively what's wrong or what they need to work on. The body is expression of our inner state. Just by watching people, I can sense things about their physical state. It's uncanny and I often surprise myself, but it makes me a good trainer. I know this comes from spending significant amounts of time in this deep, beautiful, communion.

I believe that exercise has a spiritual component. It's way of aligning with that creative force, which is the essence of the universe. Nature is always creating. There's a pushing out, an expansion; that's the nature of the Universe. Well, your spirit is your connection to that universal creative force. It shows up as this drive, this urge to create something.

I believe that exercise can unleash that creative force in you, because it gives you a sense of possibility. It gives you the ability to create on this most basic of levels—the physical body. My spirit demanded I push through my limitations, and to do that it craved some sort of discipline. I see that spirit in most bodybuilders. They're really out there pushing their personal envelopes. They're creating new ways of being. Bodybuilding/body sculpting gives you the ability to create something new, a new physiology, a new body. Bodybuilding has emboldened and empowered me to go and do more of everything else. I'm a better person for the effort and discipline.

There's a woman at my gym who has completely transformed her body. She went from weighing over 200lbs. to competing onstage as an amateur bodybuilder. Whatever was inside her that drove her to start to make the change is pretty amazing. Then, when she began to see the results, it emboldened and empowered her even further.

She's a wonderful example for others. When I don't see that creative drive in a person—when someone seems stuck in survival mode, not excited about creating—I get very concerned. If you can't go out and create your life, whether it's a new business, art, or whatever, what have you got? I think that's where exercise can yield extraordinary dividends. It can align your energies and spark the creative process, and that spills out into so many other areas of your life.

Conscious Fitness and Trauma

I see a lot of wounded people—both men and women—both in the gym and out in the world. It constantly reminds me that humans are actually very vulnerable. As my Native teachers taught, early humans felt very at risk physically because we didn't have the natural defensive equipment that many animals have. We weren't naturally endowed with fangs or claws or poisonous bites. We didn't have wings to fly away from an attacker or thick, impenetrable hides. By comparison, we were weak, so we had to rely on our wits and our ability to sense a threat (or opportunity) quickly and react. We responded by using technology to create weapons that mimic—and go way beyond—the natural defenses of animals. Although we are now the most dominant species, we still carry that ancient sense memory of vulnerability around with us today; it's buried in our subconscious: an ancient "operating system" waiting to be triggered.

We're also vulnerable psychologically, emotionally, psychically. We're social beings, so we're vulnerable to other people, to their opinions and actions. Most of us have been profoundly wounded, in one way or another. And we're naturally empathic. We feel for others, whether we acknowledge it consciously or not. That's a lot of vulnerability to carry around.

Both genders manipulate their physical beings in order not to seem so vulnerable.

Men often seek to protect themselves by developing muscles as a kind of armor; it's a way of putting up a barrier so things can't get in and hurt them as may have happened when they were children.

Many men also deny pain. Muscles create a shield and the denial of pain creates the mental illusion of invulnerability. (Unfortunately, it can also help to make us insensitive.) The denial of pain seems to be at the core of how some men view their masculinity. I've seen men continue to run every day even though they have a broken foot. It's as if they're saying to themselves, "If I'm tough, nothing can get me."

Men often seem to act as if they see their bodies as something to be used up. Many men just hurl themselves at things without regard for consequences. My friend and client, Mike, is a great example. In training him, I'll want him to push into new territory—and I'll want to hear feedback so I can gauge how it's working for him. "I want to try this with you, but I need you to let me know what you're feeling," I'll say. He'll start doing it and I'll see him wince. But instead of saying that he's experiencing some pain, he'll respond by saying, "I can do it." Yes, he may be able to do it, but I may not want him to because his body might not be ready. If that's the case, I can find another way to accomplish the goal.

My point is that men will often ignore pain. They'll push through it instead of acknowledging it. But pain, as we'll discuss in more detail in a later chapter, is actually a very important form of feedback. Pain can be "good," in that it's a sign of growth and a confirmation that you're doing the right thing. It can also be "bad," a signal to stop what you're doing immediately. Ignoring bad pain can lead to injury. The denial of pain is not a conscious approach to fitness.

Trauma can show up differently in women. Some withdraw from anything physical. I've owned several gyms, and my experience is that many women shy away from joining a co-ed gym because they're so beaten down that they feel they couldn't exercise or use their bodies in front of men. Some women shake just at the idea of joining a gym. Other women gain weight to protect themselves, particularly if they've been abused in some way. For those women, the extra padding can act as a kind of armor, providing a sense of safety.

I have some personal experience with this feeling of vulnerability. When I was about six years old, a mentally challenged neighbor molested me. There were other, similar incidents along the way as well. I don't think this is unusual. Probably more women than not have been harmed in some way: assaulted, raped, or beaten or have been victims of incest, whether they want to admit it or not. We need to acknowledge the reality that many girls and women have been hurt.

When I think about this, what comes to mind is the John Irving book, *Hotel New Hampshire*. The female character was raped, but learns to cope and eventually to heal. The words that stay with me are spoken to that character: "They got you, but they didn't get the *you* in you."

Many people—both men and women—respond to trauma by disassociating, by splitting off or removing part of themselves from themselves and from the world. When we experience trauma as a child we often feel that we don't have the right to be here on the planet, so we pull back; we split off and part of us goes somewhere else, somewhere where we feel safer.

If you've experienced trauma, exercise can help you support and strengthen the *you in you*. I know there are many women who hesitate to lift weights for fear of bulking up. But that's an unfounded fear. The best thing women can do for their bodies—and their minds and spirits—is to lift weights.

Lifting weights can help counteract and heal that sense of trauma by bringing you back into your body. It can help *ground* you in the physical realm, help you strengthen your relationship with yourself. It's not a cure-all, of course, but it can help you regain the feeling that you have a right to be here, on Earth, and in your body. When you start lifting weights, you exude something different; there's a different aura about you. It's not that what you exude isn't feminine; it's that it's not weakness.

Is that why I lift weights? Not consciously, but I do like the feeling of more power, more authority, of moving more strongly through the world that it gives me. It was very intriguing to push my body and see it, like an art piece, coming together. My upbringing conditioned me not to be seen; bodybuilding gave me a way to let myself be seen. Bodybuilding gave me permission to be present to myself. It has helped me get through my life on every level.

A lean, strong body is awesome; it feels great. When you feel a sense of control over your body, you feel you have control over your life—and that's very empowering. Today, too few of us feel that way. As a nation, I believe we've got to get stronger.

For women, especially, fitness can be a huge source of empowerment. Exercise toughens you in body, mind and spirit. When you push against something that doesn't want to move, it strengthens you. It gives you some fight. It's about recognizing that being feminine doesn't mean being weak or soft. It's about honoring the right of women to be here on Planet Earth at this time, and to show up strong no matter what.

Conscious Fitness can help both genders to center themselves. For many men, I think there's a great deal to be learned about what strength and power really are; that strength comes in many forms, not just the "macho" stereotype we've all been conditioned to buy into. It's about becoming more intimate with their bodies; it's not just about moving weight on a bar or acquiring muscles.

Conscious Fitness and Body Image

I want to talk about body image because that, to me, is another aspect of your spirit.

As I've said, my Native teachers taught that human beings love to take things to extremes. That's our tendency, so we have to monitor ourselves so that we can hold that tendency in check. We have to become especially conscious and mindful about those things that might become addictive.

With respect to our bodies, it's difficult—particularly for women, but for men, too—because all the magazines lure us in with these unattainable ideals. The women on the cover of the magazines—whether it's *Cosmopolitan* or the bodybuilding magazines—have all been digitized to perfection. We all know this intellectually, but the images still work on us subliminally.

Because of all this perceived pressure from society, some people insist on a low-fat, low-carb diet because they equate extreme thinness with health. Well, that's not so. We need a certain amount of padding. The brain is fatty, and the organs are cushioned by fat. We use fat for energy. So there needs to be a healthy level of fat in our diet. We have to see past the magazines that try to scream at you and seduce you. Thin does not necessarily mean healthy! In fact, there is a kind of syndrome known as TOFI, "thin outside, fat inside."

But we forget this and so we have a tendency to go to extremes. I've seen this happen with bodybuilders. When we're competing, we can get ourselves down below 6% body fat. That's really, really lean, by the way. Simultaneously, you're trying to maintain muscle size, so you don't want to get into a catabolic state where you're destroying muscle tissue. It's a very delicate balance—and not particularly healthy.

If you manage to achieve that for competition, then you start thinking you should be able to maintain that 6% body-fat all year-round. Well, you can't. The truth is that state is very tenuous and can only be held for a very short time. It's not logical, normal, or achievable to maintain that without doing serious damage to your body. But still, people try.

That's one kind of extreme. On the other extreme, many competitive bodybuilders will nearly starve themselves to get into competitive shape, and then binge and balloon out between competitions. That, too, is very hard on the body. I never did that. I made sure I was always getting about 2000 calories a day, and I was never more than 10-12 pounds outside my competitive weight between events. This discipline allowed me to keep competing, and I was never weak from dieting. The whole time I was competing I felt really good. I didn't let myself get out of shape too far.

So there's extremism with respect to diet and extremism with respect to exercise.

In general, the competitive bodybuilding state is neither healthy nor maintainable. It's just not normal for most people to have six-pack abs all the time.

So, if you're going to do bodybuilding as a hobby, or because you like the way it looks or makes you feel, you don't have to go to those extremes. Yes, you have to "feed the machine," *i.e.*, the body, to get what you want out of it, but don't feel you have to walk around "shredded" all the time because that is not a healthy state.

Conscious Fitness: Seeking Balance

Overdoing exercise is often a signal of underlying trauma. In my view, people who feel they have to push their bodies in these ways are trying to push something out. Athletes who are trying to push their bodies to extremes are trying to combat or push away something, instead of dealing directly with whatever it is. It's like they think they can subdue their minds by exhausting their bodies. To some extent, I've found that to be true; exercise can help quiet our over-active minds. But we can also use exercise as way to avoid important things, as a way of numbing ourselves out. Why else would you want to keep pushing through pain barriers without regard for potential injury?

If you find yourself doing this, stop and ask yourself: What am I trying to push through? Why am I doing this to my body? To my life? And how long can I sustain it?

You may find this way of thinking odd, coming from a bodybuilder. But experience has taught me that you can push through pain barriers in a damaging way or an undamaging way. There is some pain you just don't want to push through. You have to be able to sense—feel—the difference, and respond accordingly. That's why it's so important to know *your* body.

How do you keep yourself in check with regard to your exercise regimen? Just as with any sport, there are many factors that have to come together to make it happen. And we don't all have them. Although we are no longer together I was fortunate to have a supportive spouse at the time, Bill. I didn't have to work outside the home; training was my work. It had to be because it is almost a full-time job if you want to get to that level. Knowing those things, do you have the life circumstances that'll support you in a similar way? If you don't, it doesn't mean you can't do bodybuilding; it just means you're not as likely to compete at that level.

You can exercise too much. You can get addicted to it. One day, it just happens. You start striving for that perfect body and suddenly you're out of balance. I saw a lot of this when I was a professional bodybuilder. You get addicted to the way you look when you're competing, but that is an artificial state; it's not healthy for the long-term—but you can't stop. You're in trouble. So here's a word for the wise. The things to check for are the things you'd check for regarding alcoholism or any other addiction. Ask yourself: Is my exercise and diet regimen affecting my relationship and/or my work negatively? Am I going to lose my marriage because I want to be on stage? Is it affecting my money negatively? Be careful of these things and stay vigilant about it. Don't give in to it. Don't surrender your spirit. It's not about perfection, and it's certainly not just about appearance.

In sum, I see spirit and fitness, spirit and health as a very connected. I believe that feeling and being healthy feeds our spirit, and I believe that a strong spiritual foundation is essential for true health and wellbeing. The two go together; they reinforce each other. Now, I want to be clear that I'm not talking about dogma here; I'm not advocating any particular religious tradition. Given my background, that's the last thing I'd want to be doing. No. What I'm pointing to is a recognition that there is something beyond our individual existence that animates us, that gives us life, and gives life to all of the other species on Earth, and that Life Force is powerful and profoundly creative. We should be grateful for it, and we should honor it. By keeping ourselves healthy, we honor the Life Force within us.

6. The Case for Strength Training

ENTROPY HAPPENS. If you don't put new tires on your car or oil in the engine, it won't run well and it definitely won't last. The same is true for your body: If you neglect it, your body will deteriorate just as any system that isn't maintained will fall apart. Left alone, as we age our muscles have a tendency to shrink, which can lead eventually to a condition known as sarcopenia (atrophied muscles).

As we age, our metabolism also tends to slow down, beginning in our mid-20s, and we tend to gain weight. If we don't do anything to counteract these tendencies, what ensues is a "perfect storm," with the deterioration accelerating over time. According to Dr. Wayne L. Westcott, if you're inactive in your 30s and 40s, you'll lose 1/2 lb. of muscle every year. From midlife on, you'll tend to *lose 5 lbs. of muscle* while also *gaining 15 lbs. of fat* every decade.[37] That means a woman in her 60s might have 20 lbs. less muscle and 60 lbs. more fat than she did in her 20s. At this point, she may think that consuming fewer calories (dieting) is the solution. This might help her lose weight—but it won't do anything to slow the loss of muscle, which is the real root cause of the problem.

That's because lean muscle is the key to maintaining good metabolism. A toned, active muscle is like a well-tuned car engine; even when it's idle, it burns calories. In contrast, the less muscle you have, the more your metabolism slows. But, by exercising in the right way, you can slow or stop muscle loss, which, in turn, can fire up your metabolism – helping you to stay trim and feel energized and vital.

In short, *action is required*; it's not going to get better on its own, but only through effort and attention and intention. This is a message none of us want to hear—including me. I hear the screams of protest all the time. "I didn't used to have to do this!" "I used to be able eat anything I wanted!" "When I was in high school I ran five miles every day!" Great, but what are you doing now? I get it, I really do, because I'm the same as you. I want things to be easy, too. But my job in life is to take a stand for fitness, to help you understand your body's needs and help you work through your resistance, whatever it is and take action.

Now here's the most important part: **It has to be the right kind of action.** That's where strength training comes in.[38] Nothing else can take the place of strength training, whether you want to be a runner, tennis player, golfer or just a healthy person. So what do I mean by strength training? I mean *weightlifting, i.e.,* working with weights to fortify your musculature and skeletal structure.

Why Weight?

I'll say it definitively: **Weightlifting must be the basis of every fitness program.** Where once that would be a pretty radical statement, there's a lot of research now backing me up. Here's an excerpt from a recent article in *Forbes* magazine:

"Weightlifting has been controversial in the fitness industry, in medicine, and in social discourse. New scientific research on the health benefits of weightlifting however, is beginning to debunk the many myths that have undermined the positive aspects of training with weights. The studies focus on the physiology and biomechanics of strength training and bring us more evidence than ever before about what we need to do in order to be in good health and great shape through all stages of life. The evidence also recommends ways to workout with weights to achieve the best results for our own individual bodies."[39]

The Cardiovascular/Aerobic Exercise Myth

You'll often hear people say, "I run and therefore I'm fit," but it's not true—even if they look great. Their legs may be in great shape, but what about their upper body? Running alone doesn't seem sufficient to fortify the body or make it strong overall.

In fact, a commonly held belief is that fitness means doing 45 minutes to an hour or more a day of intense aerobic activity. But aerobic aka cardiovascular exercise (defined as exercise that raises your heart rate and respiration while using large muscle groups repetitively and rhythmically) *alone* is *not enough*. **Furthermore, in actuality, there are many dangers associated with doing *just* aerobic training** to the exclusion of strength training. These dangers include:

- Osteoarthritis . . . even at a younger age
- Tendonitis and other repetitive strain injuries
- Increased oxidative damage (production of free radicals)
- Susceptibility to injury and to infections
- Loss of bone density
- Depletion of lean muscle tissue - Yes, aerobic-only training actually causes you to lose muscle!
- Suppressed metabolic function[40]

In short, weightlifting (*aka* strength training) should be the foundation of any fitness program. Here's an easy way to tune into that. Remember our discussion **about the chakra system** and how the energies get increasingly denser as you move down into the physical realm? The body, being the densest form of energy, is the foundation for the other aspects of ourselves: the mental and spiritual. This follows right along with that. Since weights are dense and heavy, they should be the *base foundation* of your fitness regimen. In that way, they serve as the base foundation for your healthy life.

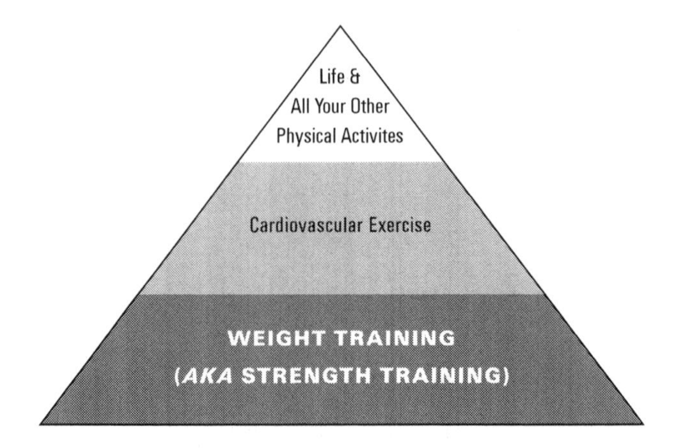

Working with weights fortifies you and makes you strong. Everything else you do should build off of that foundation, a foundation made strong through weight training. This is especially true for seniors.

Aging and the Case for Weight Training: Make Yourself "Harder to Kill"

Why are some people able to remain active and engaged well into their elder years, while others become increasingly fragile and sick? Two recent studies published in the *British Medical Journal* revealed that muscular strength is a remarkably strong predictor of mortality. "Taken as a whole, exercise has been shown to add between six and seven years to a life span — if not more." As one writer put it, "getting stronger will help you live longer" because it makes you "harder to kill."

But not all exercise is equal, he goes on to say: "Resistance training (such as lifting weights), in conjunction with high intensity workouts (like aerobics and running), is key." In sum, the scientific evidence is pointing toward weightlifting as essential to aging well. Or, as this writer put it, "Seniors need to lift weights. Actually, they *really* need to lift weights."[41]

There's nothing better than weight training to combat aging. Here's why. About a decade ago, William Evans, PhD and Irwin H. Rosenberg, professors of nutrition and medicine, respectively, at Tufts University USDA Human Nutrition Research Center on Aging (HNRCA) determine how to measure how old you are, physiologically. They published their findings in a book, *Biomarkers: 10 Determinants of Aging You Can Change.*

These biomarkers are:

1. Muscle Mass
2. Strength
3. Basal Metabolic Rate
4. Body Fat Percentage--and waist size management
5. Aerobic Capacity
6. Blood-sugar Tolerance
7. Cholesterol/HDL Ratio
8. Blood Pressure
9. Bone density
10. Ability to regulate Internal Temperature

Evans and Rosenberg also found that *strength training was the intervention that most positively affected all of those biomarkers*, a conclusion that was somewhat radical for the time.[42] They subsequently cited evidence that even people aged 84-96 who engaged in strength-training *increased their strength 50 percent in just three months* and improved their health radically. So who really knows what the limits are?

Scientific research has continued to tell us that *wisely designed and executed* strength training, aka weightlifting, has the following benefits:

- Significantly reduces co-morbidities like arthritis, diabetes, back pain, and depression;
- Reduces pain experienced by 43 percent amongst adults age 50+ (such as low back and arthritic pain), while increasing strength and performance;
- Improves balance and lowers the risk of falls by 40 percent;
- Improves bone density enough to counter the bone mass loss experienced by post-menopausal women (1 to 2 percent per year), while also improving mood and sleep;
- Leads to leaner body composition—and therefore a decrease in heart disease, as well as increased aerobic capacity;
- Increases muscle mass, which reduces age-related loss of muscle (called sarcopenia), which leads to frailty and the inability to do everyday activities;[43]
- Increases our metabolic rate, which helps to "regress obesity;"
- Keeps the brain active and the nervous system and body attuned to the coordination of movement;
- Reduces our resting blood pressure
- Increases blood sugar (glucose) control—which helps counter diabetes.[44]
- Increases gastrointestinal transit time, which is likely to reduce our risk of colon cancer;[45]
- Improves our mental health and our sex lives, keeping us more youthful.

What's the science behind this? Again, it starts with our **mitochondria**, the energy powerhouses of our cells. As we age, our mitochondria start to degrade, resulting in weaker cells and muscle fibers. We experience this as reduced endurance, strength, and function. But remember our earlier discussion of how exercise fires up our mitochondria? According to Mark Tarnopolsky at McMaster University in Ontario, **resistance-training** kick starts a process that rejuvenates our mitochondria. Tarnopolsky claims that after six months of twice weekly strength exercise training, the biochemical, physiological and genetic signature of older muscles are "turned back" by a factor of 15 to 20 years![46]

Another aspect of aging is our decreased production of telomerase, a crucial enzyme that maintains and repairs our chromosomes. When we can't produce enough telomerase, our chromosomes degrade; our genetic integrity is compromised, and so too is cellular division—leading to cell death. Again, studies indicate that **high intensity exercise** stimulates the production of telomerase.

Then there's our growth hormone. Growth Hormone (known as GH) supports the growth of tissue in the human body and can also decrease the production of fat tissue, helping us maintain favorable body composition, bone health, and general physical wellbeing. GH declines significantly as we age. (By 60, we've lost 80% of the GH we had when we were 20.) Signs and symptoms of low GH levels are increased body fat, reduced lean tissue (muscle), less energy, poor general health, and often a lack of positive wellbeing. Now there's some evidence that when you get into the four-rep range in a "big" exercise—like bench presses or squats—it signals the body to stimulate your GH. Increasing your levels of GH helps increase muscle mass, stimulates fat loss, improves skin texture and exercise tolerance, increases bone density, improves sleep quality and helps cognition.[47]

Exercise also triggers the production of antioxidants, which boosts the health of the body in general.

Our production of the hormone testosterone also decreases as we get older, resulting in a decrease in muscle and bone mass. Exercise can re-stimulate the production of testosterone, too.[48] It also results in lower levels of dangerous cholesterol.

Even more remarkable is the research that shows that resistance training can *stave off cognitive decline*. A study conducted at the University of British Columbia, involving women between the ages of 70 and 80 who were experiencing mild cognitive impairment, showed that lifting weights improved memory and staved off the effects of dementia. It also improved the participants' attention spans and ability to resolve conflicts.[49]

Psychological and Spiritual Benefits of Weightlifting

I know the idea of weightlifting seems counter-intuitive to many older people. They think it's going to hurt or they're convinced they're too old to start or they're not strong enough to do a workout. But why would they be? You've got to work out to get stronger. And I know many of us have an addiction to comfort. As we get older that can translate into a feeling that says, "I've paid my dues and I deserve to eat whatever I want." Or, "I've lost my motivation and now I'm going to play golf, or sit on the couch." Sure, we're older and more tired, but it's about not letting those excuses stop us. It's *supposed* to be a little difficult; if it's not, then we're not pushing ourselves. And isn't that the very essence of aging?

We "age," both psychologically and spiritually when we put limits on ourselves, when we stop pushing into new territory. But if we keep pushing ourselves forward, we stay younger. Evolutionarily speaking, to be alive means to keep pushing into new territory, because we don't really know what's possible or impossible.

As we age, we may forget how to do certain things, such as how to jump, but weight training can help us recover those capabilities. It will boost your coordination, your bone strength, your muscle strength, your energy, your reflexes, your balance, your vitality; it's all there when you lift weights. And it's never too late to start. Here's an example. A client, in his 60s, had a bad back that was stopping him. A year ago he would have been afraid and not attempted this, but now he's capable of doing a perfect plank pose and push-ups for 12 reps. I wish I had a video of it because he looks so strong.

The Benefits of Weight Training for Women

Let's focus on **women** for a moment. With the onset of menopause, estrogen starts to decrease and so does our supply of growth hormone. I believe, as do others, that the dramatic reduction of both estrogen and growth hormone that occurs with menopause causes accelerated aging, loss of muscle and fat accumulation. The good news is that strength training has been shown to increase our GH levels, which has a rejuvenating effect on our bones, skin and hair. However, women need more intense strength training with *less rest and more work done in a set amount of time* to raise our growth hormone above baseline.[50] Moreover, it's arguably even more important for women to lift weights on account of our higher propensity for osteoporosis.

Despite all this evidence, many women fear "bulking up," but this is a myth that needs to be put to rest. Because our bodies naturally produce more GH, we are protected from bulking up by our genetic makeup.[51]

Lifting Weights Can Lift Your Spirits

There is a subtler aspect to this, a psycho-spiritual dimension that goes beyond the physical. **Changing our body's energies can alter our souls**. Quite literally, **lifting weights can lift our spirits**. As you bring your body into proper vibrational alignment there's a resonance created that truly transforms people. I see this all the time in my clients. Let me give you an example. I'd been working with a man in his 60's (referred to in an earlier chapter). Meantime, his wife had never set foot in a gym. But, little by little, as she saw the changes in her husband—not just physical changes, but changes in the way he thought about himself—and she became intrigued enough to come in and talk with me. She was curious, but also very cautious, at least at first. She, too, was in her 60s. Tiny in stature, she'd never lifted weights before. She'd also recently undergone a laminectomy, an operation involving the removal of some of her neck bone. It was apparent when you looked at her; you could actually lay your finger in a groove in the back of her neck. She also had some lower back issues.

I evaluated her situation and told her that she needed to develop some muscle—basically, to help her hold her neck up! So we started working together. After working twice a week for three-four months, things changed dramatically. Not only does she have much stronger neck muscles, but also her entire physique has transformed. We've been doing balance work and, as a consequence, her horseback riding is getting better. And, again, the change is more than physical. It's affecting everything. Now she and he husband can speak in one voice about what's happening. They both have more confidence in all areas of their lives. It's really cool.

For women, in particular, weight training can be transformative. Weight training can teach women the importance of honoring themselves first and foremost. If, as a woman, you feel vulnerable, my advice is to get stronger. Put some muscle on you. When you push against something that doesn't want to move, like a weight, it toughens not only your body, but your mind and spirit, too. Lifting weights gives you some fight. I can't offer platitudes or secrets. *Nike*™ was right; it comes down to one thing. *Just do it.* If you need someone to help you get through that, find that person. At least give yourself a fighting chance.

I know from personal experience that weight training has many lessons to teach.

As I said, I was a very fearful child. The fear came in waves, and it still does. The fear came from the apocalyptic dogma of the Jehovah's Witnesses to which my parents subscribed so strongly. As a consequence of all of this in my early upbringing, I perceived myself as weak, and as not good at things as other kids. I was shy and held myself back.

Bodybuilding helped me transcend my fears. I was 22 when I started lifting. I began competing just 18 months later and went on to reach the top in my sport. I loved that it was something I could do by myself. I didn't have to play on a team or compete with anyone else. For me, the competitive process was internal; I only thought about my goals and how I wanted to get my body to the next point in my development. Then, when I found myself wanting to try other things, like rollerblading, mountain biking or snowboarding-even yoga—I was still afraid, afraid of failing, of injury, of being laughed at. Each time, I had to go through the whole process of trying to find my courage. Finally, I figured it out: The fears were never going to go away. There's no reasoning it out; If I wanted it bad enough, I just had to do it. Strap the skates on and go. Get on that bike. If you fall, you laugh at yourself. Everyone has to start somewhere.

Bodybuilding—lifting weights—helped me to heal in mind and spirit. I happen to have had quite a bit of drama and trauma in my early life—not as much as some people, I know, but enough. (There's really no point in comparing.) But once I found bodybuilding, I had a structure in my life that supported me. My ex-husband, a behavior modification specialist, often said that the best way to avoid a nervous breakdown is to create a structure, find some activity that you can go and do to stop the obsessive thinking that tends to take over. Lifting weights can definitely fill that bill; it's something you can do, no matter what—and it interrupts the cascade of negative thoughts. It begins to move your body's energies in a different way, in a way that helps you to get control of them so that you can manage those trauma-dramas in your life. I never did drugs or alcohol when I felt scared or overwhelmed. No, instead I'd say to myself, "I have to stop thinking about these negative things because I have to go work out." I had to refocus my energy on how the muscle felt— what I was doing/feeling in the moment. So developing muscles will benefit people in ways far beyond just improving what they look like. I'm living proof of that.

I see this all the time when I'm training people. Within the first two weeks, their visage changes. I see new muscle, but that's not the only thing. Something in their energy field changes. It brightens. It's refreshed. I've never seen it fail. Now mind you, just getting a membership in a gym doesn't do it; you actually have to come in! And, of course, any exercise of this type should be done in consultation with your doctor and under the supervision of trained professionals.

That said, a lot of people, especially women, have misconceptions about using weights and weight training. They're afraid if they use them that they'll "bulk up" in odd and unattractive ways. But a weight is just a tool. It's the way you use the tool that leads to the results you get—and you have control over that. Take Tiger Woods for example. Tiger was one of first golfers to start using weight training to improve his golf game. If you look at his body, he looks fit, but doesn't look like a bodybuilder. Yet, his use of weights has improved his game and also, more than likely, his ability to play longer because weightlifting is such a fortifier.

The Body You Want

One thing that can help you see how much control you really have over the results you can achieve is to look at examples of how different bodies look, depending on what kind of exercise they do. Look at track and field, particularly marathon runners vs. sprinters. Their big, muscular thighs are meant for explosive action. In general, sprinters' bodies are like those of a professional bodybuilder's. That's because sprinting has a lot in common with bodybuilding; both sprinters and bodybuilders go full out for short bursts. Then they rest.

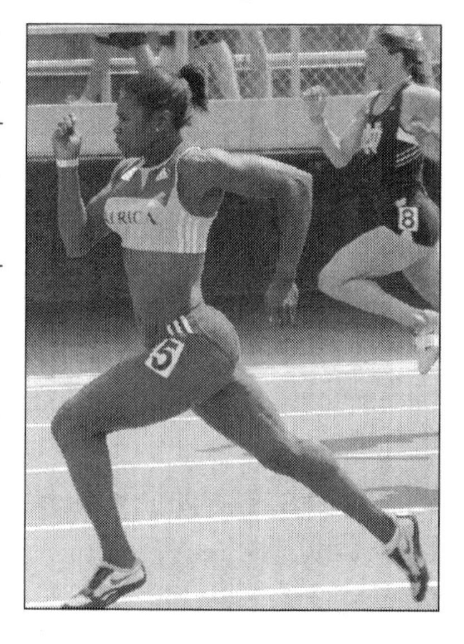

By contrast, a distance runner's body is much leaner.

Now consider power lifters and professional body builders. They both use the same tools—weights—but they achieve two completely different outcomes.

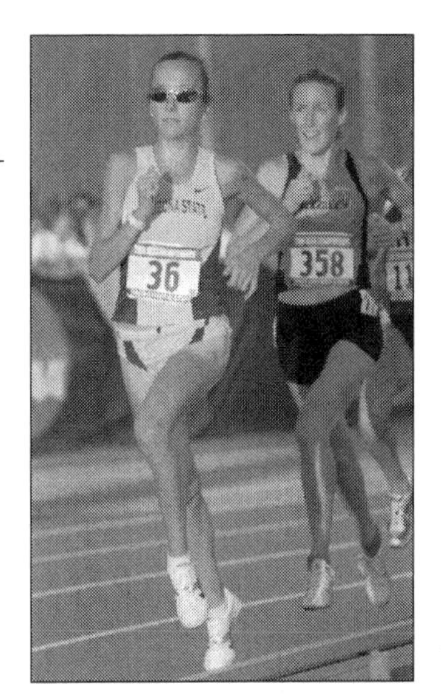

Now that we've covered the benefits of strength training, let's look at the three major types of weight/strength training you can choose from.

7. The Three Kinds of Strength Training

THERE ARE THREE different kinds of workouts that use weights, each of which yields very different results. They are:

- Power lifting
- Conditioning
- Bodybuilding/Body Sculpting

Let's do a quick tour of each. Even if you think you already know the differences, please bear with me. There are a lot of misconceptions out there.

Power Lifting

At its most basic, power lifting is about moving a weight while asking the underlying question: What 's the *most* weight I can move?

Benefits

There are benefits to controlled power lifting. It fortifies the body in a certain way, *i.e.*, it increases muscle. There's also my view that power lifting just toughens you up mentally. When you've proven to yourself that you won't collapse under a certain weight, it builds your confidence and mental toughness, and I might add, a healthy dose of self-esteem—even if you haven't done it for a while. For example, I believe I could probably do a 200-lb. bench press if I worked toward it again. I have no doubt that knowledge strengthens my sense of personal power.

Downside

Taken too far, there is a risk of injury as you're overloading the skeletal structure.

The Conditioning Workout

A conditioning workout differs from power lifting in that it is typically more of a *full body workout*, which power lifting typically is not.

A conditioning workout might look like this: Doing a jumping jack, and then dropping to the ground to do a push up. Then popping back up to do another jumping jack. Knees in, knees back. Feet up, feet back. So it's an all-over conditioner. Conditioning workouts also move relatively quickly. There's little resting between sets, if at all.

In a typical conditioning workout, you may be doing plyometrics, which is basically, in the very simplest terms, jumping up onto something or down off something. The benefit of a plyometric exercise is that muscle fibers react differently when they're stopping motion with that kind of force. They develop differently.

A conditioning workout will also use weights, but in a different way from power lifting. Our bodies are held upright through a system of tension whereby one muscle pulls and another pushes. A muscle that works opposite another is called "antagonistic." In a conditioning workout you typically move from one body part to an antagonistic body part with little or no rest.

There's a buzzword that's gaining traction now in the fitness trade: "functional training." It's really just another way of talking about a conditioning workout; all training is "functional." So, if you hear that term, don't let it confuse you. The fitness industry is always looking for a "better mousetrap," a new way to package things.

Benefits

Conditioning workouts are really great for overall fitness. I run my clients through them often. They're also really great for improving coordination and proprioception, which is your sense of balance, particularly your sense of where you are in space. Because you're moving quickly in a conditioning workout, you have to train yourself to be aware of yourself and your surroundings. As your muscle tires from rapid movement, you can get sloppy and forget form.

The Downside

A conditioning workout is great for general fitness, but it's not specifically geared toward muscle shaping. That's not to say that you won't create more muscle by engaging in a conditioning workout, but the goal isn't to sculpt your body *per se*.

Conditioning workouts are really great for people who are not being drawn to changing their bodies in a very specific way and who are more attracted to endurance as a goal.

Bodybuilding

Bodybuilding is about taking control of your body and changing it based upon your vision. At its core, bodybuilding is about *breaking down muscle and then rebuilding it in such a way that the muscle reconstitutes itself differently, as more defined and more powerful.* The technical term for how we build muscle is "hypertrophy."

I know there are some misconceptions about bodybuilding and that therefore the term "body sculpting" might be more acceptable.

In fact, I struggled with what term to use for this book, but decided that we shouldn't run from the term because it is really so empowering *to build your body.* That said, I want to separate competitive bodybuilding from bodybuilding in general. Building muscle by using bodybuilding techniques does not mean *over-developing* your muscles, which is what you see when you look at a competitive bodybuilder. That only comes with taking bodybuilding to extremes, which is not the intention here. The focus in this book is on using the techniques of bodybuilding to achieve the results *you* want. Remember, you're always in control of *your* fitness regimen. It's *your* workout; it's about meeting *your* goals, and you're always in charge of your chosen level of musculature.

So, if you're trying to strengthen your muscles and re-shape your body—as are most people who work out—you *are* bodybuilding.

Benefits

I think there's nothing better than my bodybuilding techniques for helping the layperson start to understand his or her body. And, unlike many other sports, the great thing about bodybuilding is that you can start at any age and still get really proficient at it. For example, we have a gentleman in our gym who started lifting when he was in his 80's. And he arrived with numerous physical problems from cardiac issues and the subsequent problems associated. He is now bench pressing 135lbs. for four or so reps and has even changed his gait and overall health. He SHINES! In sum, it's never too late to start. Are there any downsides to bodybuilding? No, not if done properly.

Three Types of Strength Training Compared

Power lifting, conditioning training, and bodybuilding workouts are all hard workouts, and all are valid, but they differ in some significant ways. First, the goals are different. The goal of power lifting is to develop your overall strength. Conditioning workouts are aimed at improving one's endurance, and the goal of bodybuilding is muscle definition.

Because the goals are different, there's a real significant difference between how power lifters and bodybuilders work with weights. In power lifting, your focus is on lifting the maximum possible weight. Therefore, a power lift typically involves *multiple joints*. It's the use of multiple joints (and multiple muscle groups) that enables you to lift a heavy weight. In contrast, bodybuilding involves focused concentration on a single muscle (or group of muscles) during a set. For example, when you're doing a compound exercise (such as a bench press) to bodybuild, your goal is to focus is on a single muscle, *i.e.,* your pecs alone, because you want to use the lift to develop that particular muscle. Focusing on a single muscle takes much more concentration than doing the same exercise as a power lift. Can you see why?

Similarly, when doing a squat with the specific intention of bodybuilding, you could narrow down your focus to your quads, glutes or hamstrings. This technique, called "muscle isolation," is the key to creating muscle definition. Because you're trying to isolate a single muscle you won't be able to lift as much weight when you bodybuild as you can when you power lift, but your lifts will be much more targeted, and you'll create more muscle definition in that particular muscle. Again, it depends upon your goals.

Certain exercises, such as a bench press, can be done either to power lift or to bodybuild, depending upon whether or not you focus on a single muscle or muscle group. For example, when a bench press is done as a power lift you employ *all* your available resources—your chest, shoulders, triceps and your back—because your goal is to lift the most weight you can. Likewise, when you do a squat as a power lift you recruit your entire core, quads, glutes, hamstrings and calves.

But when you're doing a bench press to **bodybuild**, your goal is to focus on a single muscle, such as your pecs alone, because you want to use this lift to develop that particular muscle. This takes much more (pared down) concentration. So, when you do a squat to bodybuild, you focus on either your quads, glutes or hamstrings.

Because you're trying to isolate a single muscle, you won't be able to lift as much weight when you bodybuild as you can when you power lift—but your lifts will be much more targeted. We'll talk about muscle isolation in-depth in later chapters.

Here's a precaution that follows from the distinction between power lifting and bodybuilding: Single joint movements should never be done with "power," *i.e.*, with maximum weight, because you run the risk of overloading your muscles, which can result in injury. A **bicep curl,** for example, is a one-joint movement, meaning you primarily use your bicep to move the weight. Therefore, this exercise should *never* be done with maximum weight, *i.e.*, one rep, max.

With respect to pacing, power lifting has a lot in common with bodybuilding. In power lifting, you rest between sets, *i.e.*, you do a set of squats and then sit down for a few minutes to recover so you can do the next one to maximum effort. So, too, in bodybuilding, you take a moderate amount of time to rest in between sets: maybe a 2-4 minutes. Your heart rate will be high during a set, but then you have period of recovery. In a conditioning workout, however, you move rapidly from one thing to next, with little or no rest; you keep your heart rate high throughout. Therefore, it's more endurance-based.

	PRIMARY GOAL	FOCUS	TYPICAL MOVEMENT	PACING
POWER LIFTING	Developing overall strength	Lifting maximum weight	Compound (*i.e.*, multiple joints)	Rest between sets
CONDITIONING	Endurance	Working entire body all at once	Compound	Little or no rest between sets
BODYBUILDING	Muscle growth & definition	Striving for muscle isolation	Single or compound	Rest between sets

If you're new to fitness, I suggest trying each out for a period of time, and noticing what your body might take to. Notice how different they feel. Experiment and observe. Also, when you first begin it's good to do *compound* movements, so power lifting is a good place to start. Then, if you've been doing the same thing for a while, mix it up. Create that surprise for your body. If you've been doing bodybuilding, do some power lifting. Bring in the conditioning element, too: Try doing all your sets in 45 minutes. Or even combine the techniques, within reason. The only rule is: there are no rules.

In time, it would be nice to bring all elements in at various times to keep your workout very well rounded. But, at first, do whatever gets you into the gym. Above all: ***Don't do somebody else's workout.*** Do what you enjoy doing. If you enjoy pushing a lot of heavy weight around and you know how to do it, great! Do what excites you and gets you to the gym!

Strength Training: The Four Foundational Exercises

Whether you choose to focus on power lifting, conditioning, or bodybuilding, these four exercises are foundational. As I said, it's best to begin with *compound exercises,* and that's what these all are. Compound exercises, by definition, require several joints and muscles, all working synergistically. No matter how you approach them, these core movements fortify the body in a unique way. Compound lifts trigger the release of two of the most crucial elements—testosterone and growth hormone (GH)—because so much of your musculature is being called upon. They also work the cardio-vascular system. I believe that everyone should start with these exercises, assuming they're physically capable. Get these down, get them right, and keep doing them!

1. Bench press with barbell

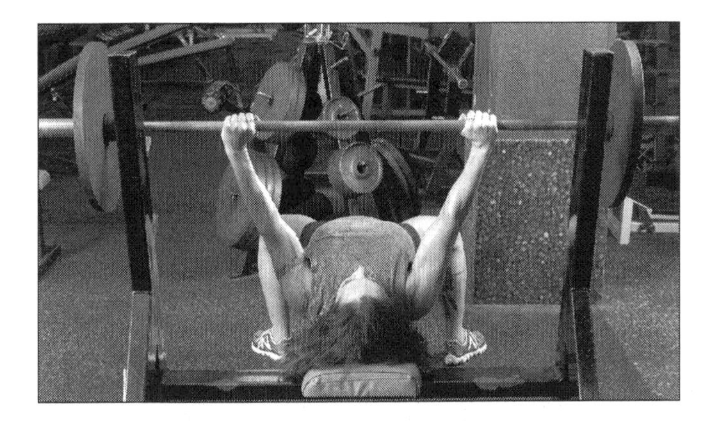

This exercise is a great all-around mass, strength and confidence builder.

2. Free Bar Squat –

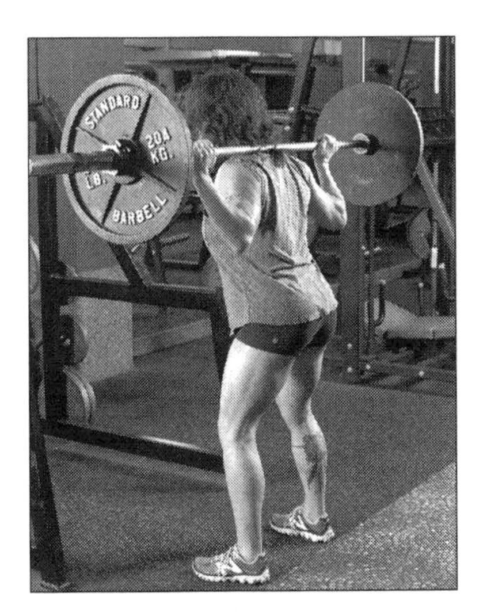

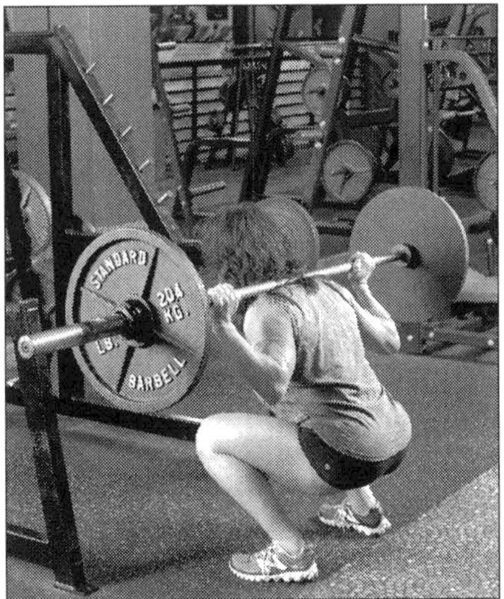

This exercise uses 70% of the muscles in your body. That's a whole lot of engagement. Therefore this exercise gives you "a lot of bang for your buck."

3. Dead Lift

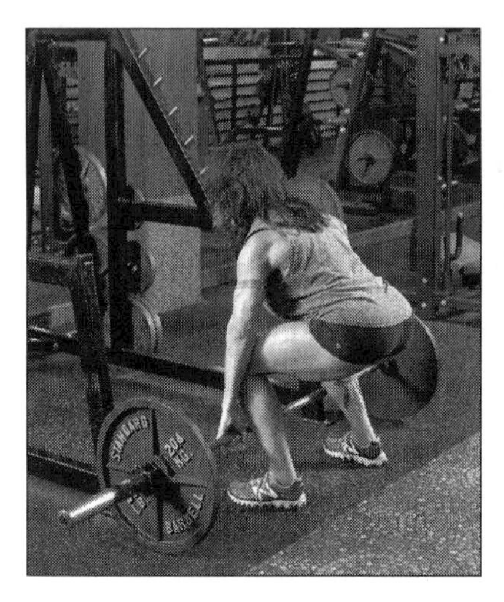

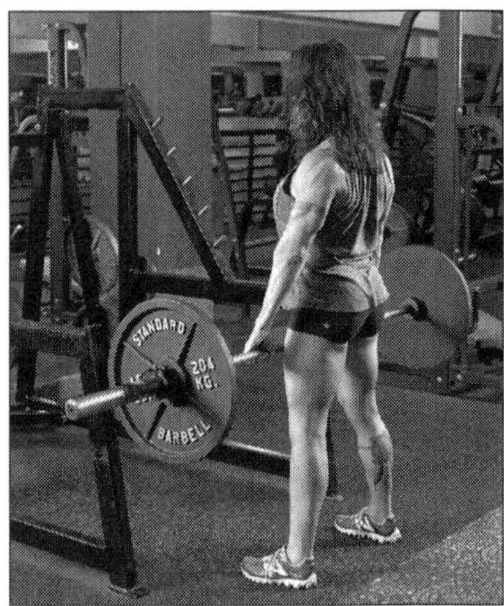

Pulling a bar from ground up, this exercise uses you arm and leg muscles plus all the muscles of your back.

4. The Pull-Up

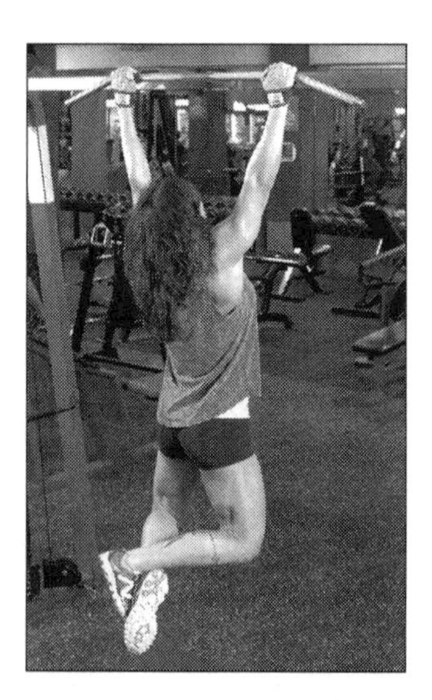

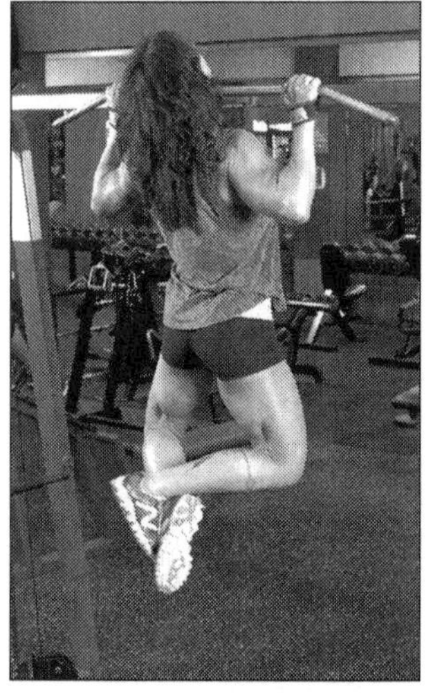

This exercise recruits many muscles in the upper body; it's a great core activator. It builds strength. And it's darn impressive!

These four exercises will build both strength and confidence. They are major muscle recruiters. They're fortifiers of both body and mind, and they provide a baseline foundation for your workout. They'll make you stronger—quickly—and then you can branch off of those. They should be the foundation for everything else you do.

Don't let anyone scare you away from them by convincing you they're dangerous. So is driving, but we still do it. We just learn how to do it safely first. The same applies to these exercises. You must learn to do these four exercises *properly*, so seek professional guidance, and then continue to do them—for years, if not forever.

Getting Started with Weight Training

A combination of free weights and machines is the best, because there are benefits to both. I encourage you to learn to work with free weights. Free weights require concentration to maintain balance and coordination. That means you really should get some instruction. If you can't afford a personal trainer right away, you can start with machines. A machine requires a lot less concentration because it does a lot of the balancing for you. But the trade-off is that you can potentially become less body-literate. You don't learn to sense and do certain things because the machine is doing it for you. You may not pay sufficient attention to your symmetry. For example, if I'm doing a chest press in a machine I might be pushing more with my left than right side. I may not realize that I'm very lopsided because the weight is still going to come along in an even way. With a free weight, however, my lop-sidedness would be more noticeable because I can see that the bar is uneven.

For a lot of people, being in machine gives them more leeway to blank out and just count reps. It's easier to drift. But when I work with free weights, I know that if I don't concentrate on what I'm doing, I'm going to feel that bar tilt and become aware of the imbalance. Plus, machines aren't totally safe either; if you don't know what you're doing—you can get hurt pretty easily—but at least you'll have a diagram on the machine to help you.

In general, though, machines force you into a certain plane—they make you hold that angle, for the most part. Quite often if someone has an injury, it's better to use free weights because they allow the body to travel in a plane more suitable to getting around their injury.

So, in sum, there are benefits to both. But if I could only use one, it would definitely be free weights because they involve more of me. **Both muscle and mind are involved; more muscle fibers are incorporated to maintain balance and coordination.**

Now that we've established the importance of weight training and you understand some of the basics, let's talk about **how my Conscious Fitness approach can be applied to strength training in order to help you maximize your workout.**

8. Conscious Fitness

THE HEART OF THE TECHNIQUE

Maximizing your Workout: Conscious Fitness as a Foundation for All Weight/Strength Training

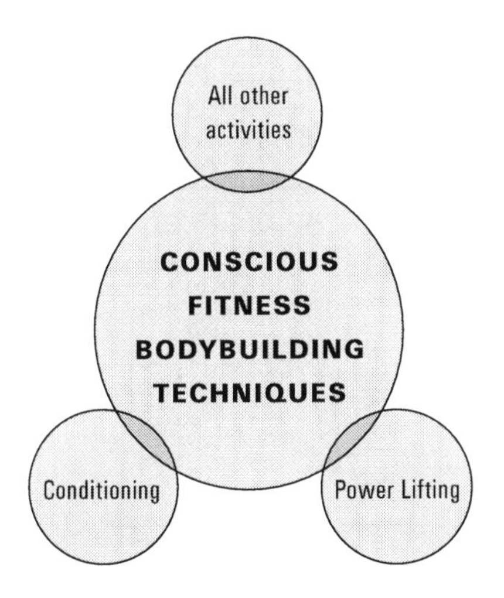

My Conscious Fitness techniques grew out of bodybuilding. However, they provide a strong foundation for *any* kind of weight training, including power lifting and conditioning. I say this for three reasons:

- *Consciousness is the key to staying safe.* Someone who's trained in my approach will be less injury-prone because they're more aware, and in communication with their body on a consistent basis.

When doing a conditioning workout, for example, you're likely to tire quickly because you're not resting between sets. As everyone knows, when we're tired, we tend to get more mindless about what we're doing; we can get sloppy and make mistakes. That's the recipe for injury. For example, if you're doing a cross-fit workout (*i.e.,* a bunch of exercises, timed), and you're racing against the clock, how mindful can you really be? That's why we're seeing lots of injuries in cross-fit now. It's highly competitive, but where is your consciousness? Is it focused on the clock? Is it distracted by someone else's performance? If you practice my Conscious Fitness approach, you'll be less likely to let your mind drift, and that will make you safer.

The same goes for power lifting. The more conscious you are as you lift, the more likely you are to be in control of the weight—and that means fewer injuries. If you practice my conscious approach to strength training—which involves learning some bodybuilding techniques, such as how to isolate a muscle, how to command a set of muscles on demand—you're likely to be a lot safer, regardless of whether you do a power lifting or conditioning workout because you'll know how to command your body in a brand new way.

- Not only will your workout be safer, it will be much *more effective and efficient*. You'll know how to command your body in a brand new way.
- Thirdly, I think there's nothing better than these techniques to help you develop an intimate relationship with your body.

So let's dig in.

At the core of my Conscious Fitness approach lies this principle:

- *The goal in each exercise is to* ***isolate and focus on working a specific muscle*** *while simultaneously* ***calming the rest of your body****.*

This is the most efficient and effective way to develop muscle and strengthen your body. Interestingly, there was mention of muscle isolation in the bodybuilding world, but any understanding of what that meant seemed rather superficial. Ironically, I didn't discover this principle through bodybuilding, but through something else entirely.

Discovering the Principle of Muscle Isolation

When I was participating in bodybuilding competitions, there were always three scored rounds.

The first round was about evaluating the symmetry of your body. Each contestant would do quarter turns in groups of 4-5 in front of a panel of judges who examined each of us to get an overall sense of how we were put together. They were especially looking to assess how evenly developed we were from back to front and from top to bottom.

Second came the muscularity round. In this round, we came out in groups of 4-5 and did compulsory poses. We'd perform side-by-side so the judges could compare our muscularity. What did each of us look like in a front double bicep pose, for example?

The third round was a free-form posing round. Each of us had 60 seconds to go through a choreographed posing routine unaccompanied by music. (Later that evening, after all the judging had taken place, we'd perform another routine before an audience: an additional ninety-second posing round set to our choice of music.)

This third round was hugely important. If you have a great routine, it gives you chance to influence judges in more subjective, emotional ways. A great routine is one that hides your flaws and brings out your best parts.

Believe it or not, the third round was the hardest in the whole competition for me. And the evening show, even though it wasn't being judged, was terrifying. It was much harder than anything I'd ever done in the gym. Static posing was much easier for me than setting a routine to music and choreographing it. I'd never performed on stage before and I knew I didn't move gracefully.

I knew I needed help, and help arrived in a somewhat unexpected package, as help often does. One day the summer before my next competition, my new next-door neighbor came over to introduce herself. Her name was Deborah Palesch, and on that day she came by dressed in high heels and a bikini. Physically, Deborah was tiny and curvy, and her personality was very outgoing. She was larger-than-life, and she had a way of looking at you that cut right through to the heart of things. In short order, Deborah revealed that she had danced with Royal Winnepeg Ballet and knew a few things about performing on stage. Something clicked. Although I'd just met her, I found myself telling her how difficult performing on stage was for me. She replied that if I was going to be on stage, I had to develop stage presence, which comes from gaining confidence in your technique and your movement.

I was scared to death, but I had to do something, so I asked her to help me with choreography. Deborah and I then began to work together on choreographing my routines. It was a very interesting collaboration because she knew nothing about bodybuilding and I knew nothing about dance. So I'd have to show her poses and together we'd string them together by putting in the conjunctions. She could even come up with poses because it's all art form; it's moving sculpture. The only question was: How can I show my body in the best light while also giving an artistic performance?

Ballet is one of the most difficult art forms. Though ballet dancers may appear delicate or even fragile, they are remarkably disciplined, strong and resilient; battered, bruised, they have the fortitude to remain elegant through it all. My experience with ballet helped me not to shy away from physical discomfort or suffering; I learned to stay with pain longer, and that helped me develop a sense of presence that translated to the stage.

At the very beginning of our collaboration, Deborah suggested I take one of her beginner ballet classes—which I did. She just neglected to mention that the class was full of six-year-olds!

So I started studying ballet—the only adult in a class full of kids. All the little girls would giggle at me, but that was actually really great because it made me laugh at myself. In that class I could set aside my fears of being judged and just be in my own little world. But I was watchful, and this is how I made one of my most important discoveries.

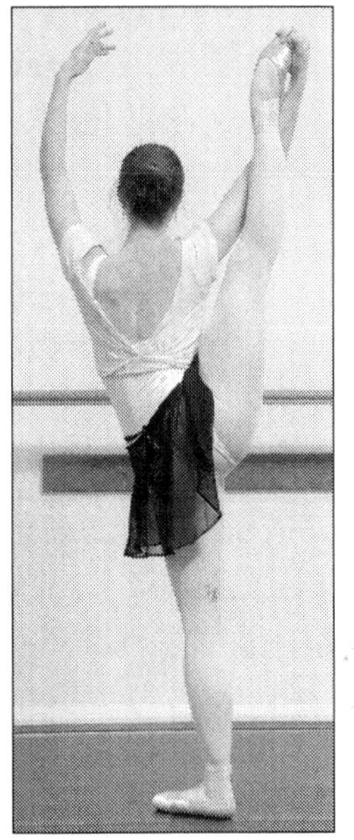

Through ballet, I saw that it was possible to lift your leg in the air above your head without shifting your hips, while still keeping them level—as if your hips weren't connected to your leg at all. I was amazed. How on earth was that possible?

In seeking to understand this, I discovered an underlying principle behind the beauty of many ballet moves: when there is *a lifting up and away from, there is also simultaneously a grounding down.* You push down on one body part at the same time as you push up with another. Doing this requires you to *isolate* one part of your body from the other parts that normally move with it.

Once I figured this out, I was absolutely taken with these two principles: *isolation* and *opposition.* Soon after, the thought dawned on me that these two principles could be applied to bodybuilding. And with that, the world broke open.

This collaboration was a tremendous success! Not only did ballet help me do well in the posing round—and therefore win competitions—but it also opened my eyes to these principles. Most people would probably reject the idea that ballet could be relevant to bodybuilding, but I'm forever grateful to it for awakening me to the isolation technique. Sometimes the conventional wisdom isn't wisdom—it's just conventional.

The Foundational Principles of Conscious Bodybuilding

In this section, I'll talk more about isolation and opposition, the two principles that lie at the core of my Conscious Fitness approach.

Muscle Isolation

Muscle definition is very important in competitive bodybuilding. Muscle definition comes from the work you do to differentiate one muscle from another. When I was competing, I knew that the more separation between my muscles I achieved, the better I'd look on stage. That's because professional bodybuilding deals in illusion: the more defined your muscles, the bigger they seem, and the better your chance of winning!

Muscle differentiation is very visually appealing. This explains why just adding a little muscle to one's frame creates an effect that is just gorgeous.

After my exposure to ballet, I began to realize that I could take the concept of isolating a body part even further: If I wanted to build a certain muscle, *I needed to isolate it and move it by itself*—without engaging any other muscle to help it move. (Of course in reality this isn't entirely possible, but I wanted to use that idea to increase the availability of the muscle I was focusing on, while simultaneously quieting to a mere whisper, the muscles I didn't want to engage.) Over time, I developed the concept of muscle isolation into a key aspect of my approach to bodybuilding/sculpting, with remarkable results. This principle lays the foundation for everything else.

The most efficient way to define your muscles is to focus on working each muscle by itself, in isolation from all other muscles. So, **muscle isolation is the key to bodybuilding.** Muscle isolation means that your focus and intention should be aimed at developing *one particular muscle.*

This is very different from the approach you take in compound exercises such as those we discussed in the last chapter. Compound exercises, by definition, require several joints and muscles, all working synergistically. For example, if you do a pull-down or pull up exercise, you're using the muscles of the back, your rear delts, biceps and incidentally, the forearms. These muscles are all functioning in a complementary fashion. Similarly, if you're rowing, you're using your back and biceps; you're using complementary muscles. HOWEVER, for the purpose of bodybuilding/body sculpting, you want to minimize the involvement of other muscles. For example, in that pull-up, you want to try to quiet the involvement of the biceps as much as possible, allowing the back to do all the work, because there are more efficient ways to work the biceps. You want to isolate each muscle as much as possible, and *use only that muscle to perform the exercise*. A **bicep curl,** for example, is not a compound exercise. It's a one-joint movement because I'm only using my bicep to move the weight, nothing else.

Compound exercises are great fortifiers but, for the purpose of bodybuilding/body sculpting, you want to focus on a single muscle and minimize the involvement of other muscles. You want to isolate each muscle as much as possible, and *use only that muscle to perform the exercise*. Again, to achieve maximum muscle definition and strength as efficiently as possible, your goal is to completely isolate a muscle so it alone is doing the work of the exercise—while simultaneously limiting the participation of every other muscle.

Now, you ask, is this really possible? No, but that's the ideal. Any exercise physiologist will tell you that, so long as multiple joints are in action, multiple muscles are in play. While that is true, we can learn to develop the ability to isolate the muscle to a greater degree than we normally would. That's the feeling you're going for. And the closer you get to accomplishing that, the more efficient your workout, and the more muscle you'll build, quickly. When you understand the benefits of muscle isolation, you can approach your exercises much more intelligently. You'll begin to develop an intuitive, felt body sense of what you're doing, and avoid the mistakes so common to folks who don't understand the underlying relationship between the exercise and the muscle.

Here's an example. Let's say you want to do a bench press with the intention of developing your pectoral muscles. If you want to use the bench press to build your pectoral muscles in the most efficient way possible, you have to make every effort to *isolate* your pecs and use *only* your pecs to move the weight. In other words, you don't want to use your shoulder or arm muscles at all. (That means that if your intention was to do a pec workout, and you wake up with sore shoulders the next day, that would be a sign that you didn't practice muscle isolation.)

When you lift to develop your pecs, the conscious bodybuilding questions to ask yourself are: Can I use *only* my pecs? To what extent can I "shut down" my shoulder muscles (deltoids) and triceps so that I'm only using my pecs to lift the weight? Now, that's a very difficult thing to do because your pecs are intimately connected with your deltoids. Some will say you just can't move your pecs independently from your deltoids. But you can. Not *entirely*, of course, but very close. And that's what you're aiming for.

Here's another example. The behind-the-neck press exercise is supposed to work your shoulder muscles. But when I observe people doing this exercise I frequently see guys arching their backs and bringing their butts to the front tip of the seat. What they don't realize is that the reason they're arching their back is to engage the chest muscles in helping their shoulders with the lift--probably so that they can lift more weight. The problem is that this posture is useful for almost everything else *except* working your shoulders, and the exercise has now become an incline chest press. This is typical when someone doesn't understand the benefits of muscle isolation—and doesn't really understand their muscles.

Along with knees, shoulders get hurt all the time. It's easy to see why if you look closely at the musculature of the shoulder. The three muscles that make up the shoulder are all short and narrow, each not very big, relatively speaking. The shoulder is actually rather delicate.

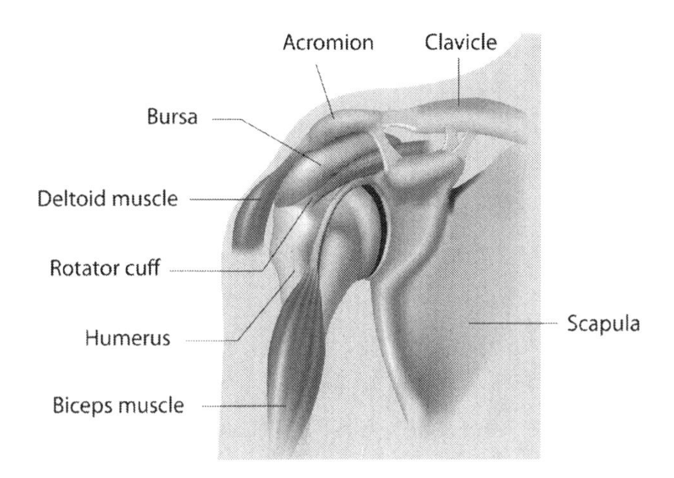

How much weight do you think you can actually push with those muscles alone? Not very much. So if you're too ambitious with the amount of weight you want to lift, chances are you're employing other muscles as well as momentum and explosiveness. In sum, if you're lifting 225 lbs. behind your neck, you're probably not using as much of your shoulder muscles as you think because you just can't lift that much weight without using other muscles; your shoulder just doesn't have the mass to lift that on its own. This is another reason to know your musculature: so you can see more clearly what you're asking of your body. In this case, you're asking a lot of a small area of muscle and, unless you want to incorporate other muscles, you need to adjust accordingly.

To remedy this problem with the behind-the-neck press, I tell folks to bring their entire spine *into the bench*—to feel each vertebra touching the bench—and drop the collarbones slightly. This will shift the burden of the lift to their shoulders, which is where they actually want it.

When they do that, the weight just stops dead because now they're no longer incorporating the muscles of the chest to help them lift it; they're feeling what they can actually lift with their shoulder muscles alone—and it's nowhere near the same. So then I tell them to cut the amount of weight they're trying to lift in half. If they were trying to lift 190, I tell them to bring it down to 95 lbs. They'll see then that even that relatively low weight might be a struggle because they've *finally isolated their shoulders*, and shoulders are actually a small muscle group.

Once you're able to work successfully with the muscle isolation technique, the results come quickly, and the effect is quite astonishing! But there's no denying that learning how to isolate your muscles takes a bit of time. The first several times you try, it might seem like you're lost. I still have to for look for it; it's a lifelong search, but here's a metaphor that might help. In my experience, it's like knowing you want to get from where you are now to a destination off in the distance, and in between is a tall, overgrown field. The weeds are so tall that you can't see your destination, so you don't know exactly where it is. You just know it's out there, somewhere, and that you've got to cross this unknown territory to get there. The first time through, it's going to be tough to find your way. You don't even have a clear idea of where you're going, so you 're tramping down weeds, feeling lost and frustrated, until finally you stumble upon a sensation that tells you "Oh, this might be where I was trying to go!" It feels different; it feels right. You've started to experience true muscle isolation. Yes!

The, the next time you try, it'll be a little easier. You may only get there in a really zigzag pattern, but you have a better feel for the goal, and you can follow the trail a little bit better. By the third, fourth, or fifth time, that path is beginning to be well worn, so it's much easier to travel. But you still have to use energy to get there. You still have to focus. It still requires high level of concentration because you're trying to build a new neurological pathway. Think back to a time when you had to learn something brand new. With time and effort, didn't you become more proficient?

It's not about the Weight

Obviously, you can move more weight if you involve all the muscles in your shoulders, arms and chest rather than just using your pecs, but effective bodybuilding/sculpting is ***not about the weight.***

It takes a while to understand this underlying principle. Most people who lift weights—including myself—get fixated on the number: Can I lift 100 lbs.? 150? 225? We just love those big numbers on the end of the bar! This goes for young males, especially. But the irony is that *fixating on the number actually results in a less sculpted body.*

If you've been lifting weights for a while, you'll feel like you're stepping backward a bit when you first begin to work with muscle isolation. The reason is straightforward. The more you isolate a muscle, the less perceived strength you'll seem to have when you lift. This is because you're working with one major muscle, and you're not incorporating the other muscles around it to help.

This brings us to another one of my principles: *weight is always relative*. Remember, for an ant, ten pounds is really heavy. It's not about the number on the weight; that's actually irrelevant. Your muscle doesn't care; it only knows whether a weight *feels* heavy or light.

Yes, you can focus on lifting a lot of weight to get a body like a power lifter, but you'll have a greater potential of hurting yourself. Or, you can start isolating your muscles—which means you can only lift so much weight—but you'll get a much more toned and sculpted body as a result. And you're much less likely to injure yourself, which means longevity in the sport and a healthy, amazing physique for many years.

Opposition

Conscious bodybuilding/sculpting is all about working with opposites. In any bodybuilding exercise—that is, any exercise in which the goal is to build muscle—*there have to be two things happening in opposition.* This is a variation of the core concept of *lifting up while grounding down.*

To derive the most benefit from any exercise, you need to ground down as you're lifting up.

This means that, no matter what muscle you're focused on developing, **you want to create a situation where one part is going up while**

the other part is not only stable, it's actually going down. When one muscle is flexing, there's simultaneous subtle movement in the opposite direction. That's the principle of opposition; you have to have something to leverage against to get the benefit of the push or pull.

Let's look at an example. Say you want to do a shoulder press. In this exercise, you're pushing up with your shoulder muscle. Great. Now, think for a moment: What could you do to introduce opposition into that exercise?

Here's what I do: Simultaneous to my shoulder muscle going up, I'm mentally taking my shoulder blades and zipping them down my spine. As I do so, my scapulae (shoulder blades) get pushed down. In short, my shoulders are raising a weight while my scapulae are actually moving the opposite way! This creates the opposition that leads to building muscle.

Here's another example: In the bench press, you're isolating your pectoral muscles as much as possible; they're the muscles you're going to use to lift the weight. So, as you're lifting with your pecs, what do you simultaneously ground down? In a bench press, push the tips of your scapulae down. There's a tendency for the scapulae to peel away from the bench as you lift the bar, but if you can learn to push down with your scapulae concurrently, you'll derive the most benefit.

In sum, to do a bench press properly, two things should be happening at the same time: you're raising the bar up with your pectoral muscles—AND you're also pushing your scapulae back, into the bench. By the way, it's not a super-hard push; it's more a *grounding down*.

Working with opposites catalyzes the muscle-building process and produces the best results. That said, it requires more control because it's more complex—but it's also much more effective than standard weightlifting. This general principle applies to all muscle-building exercises. It's one of the core principles of Conscious Bodybuilding/Sculpting. In fact, we become more conscious by asking ourselves the question: *How can I build opposition into this exercise?*

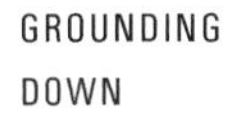

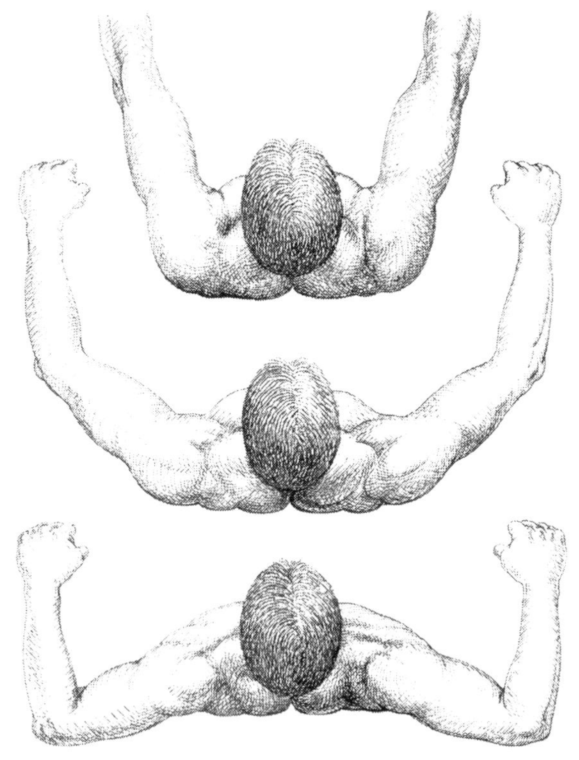

Mastering Muscle Isolation through Hypno-Fitness

Once I realized the importance of muscle isolation, my task was to learn how to do it. As I said, there was talk about "muscle isolation" in the bodybuilding world, but nobody really knew how to master it. I took that as a challenge.

Muscle isolation is like raising a single eyebrow. Before you can raise your eyebrow you have to know how to *find* the muscle that raises it. So, I began looking to *feel* each individual muscle that I wanted to work. In time I took that even further, looking to feel each *fiber* of a muscle. But in the beginning, muscle isolation was very challenging. The Native wisdom I'd learn taught me that all our body parts are separate, and yet supremely collaborative. By asking a muscle to stand alone, I was trying to peel away that collaboration in some respects.

I began to sense there was one more piece to the puzzle: I needed to **calm every other aspect of my body but the one I was working**. If I could do this it would help me to further individuate muscles.

I also needed to quiet my mind. To that, I drew on what I learned in hypnosis.

As I began to differentiate my muscles, I started becoming more intimate with them. Using the isolation principle I learned from ballet **combined with hypnosis**, I got to the point where I could *communicate* mentally with my musculature.

When my mind was quiet, I found I could actually have "respectful conversations" with these different aspects of my body. That built upon what I learned from my Native teachers. As I said, they taught that each muscle and bone, the blood, internal organs, etc., was a distinct entity with its own essence. They taught that it was important to show respect for each aspect of our bodies because these parts all served each of us; they were, in fact, allies.

In time, I began to realize that my body responded when I came from this respectful place, and I could actually create powerful alliances with my different muscles. It's hard to describe, but I call it "making deals." For example, I could ask a specific muscle do just one more curl or bench press, promising that it could stop after that—and the muscle responded!

This is very internal work, and it's really hard to do. Just ask any of my clients! You need all your powers of concentration. That's why you have to shut off the "monkey mind" and be quiet.

Now that we've laid the broad foundation, I'd like to take you on a step-by-step journey through all the steps of my Conscious Fitness conscious approach, integrating body, mind and spirit,

9. Conscious Fitness Step-by-Step

PREPARATION

AS WE'VE SAID, strength training is essential to fitness, and my **conscious fitness bodybuilding** techniques should be a part of any workout because they provide a foundation for everything else.

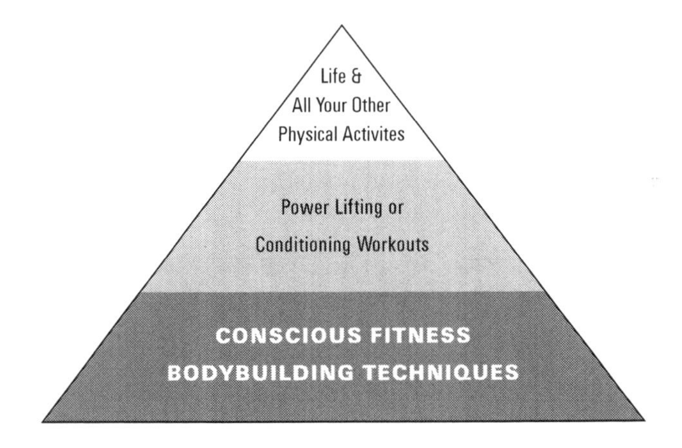

Benefits of My Conscious Fitness Approach

We're all very busy, and it's not always easy to find time to get to the gym. Therefore, you want to maximize your time there. You want to get **the most efficient workout** you can. That's what my approach provides.

Another very important benefit of my approach is that you're **less likely to suffer an injury**. Because you're not overloading the muscle, because you're not trying to move the weight at all costs, you're more stable—and safe. Also, injuries tend to happen when you move quickly. So, if you move more deliberately, with conscious intent, you're much less likely to get injured. And finally, you're so focused and aware that you can stop if you sense an injury about to happen.

For example, one time I was doing what you call a "skull crusher," a triceps exercise that involves bringing the bar down to my forehead. I was coming down so slowly, with so much concentration and control, that I was actually able to feel the muscle fibers in my triceps. All of a sudden, I felt those fibers over-stretch. It was almost like an audible sound, I heard something like "eeh," repeated three times, as if someone were plucking guitar strings. I knew something was wrong, so I immediately called to my spotter. "Take it, take it, take it!" My spotter took the bar. The next day I had a little pain and a quarter-size bruise, which meant I tore some fibers, but I was so controlled that I was able to stop before I did any serious damage. Many guys, however, will tend to keep going rather than stop at the first sign. If they keep going they can tear the muscle or tear the tendon off the bone. I've seen it happen. But because I was going so slow and constantly checking all the while, I felt it starting to go and I stopped in time. That's the difference that being conscious can make. It's almost like being able to slow down time.

A third benefit is that you'll be **developing the muscle in a more complete and well-rounded way**. That's because you'll be going through full ranges of motion rather than doing short, snappy movements (where you may not be going all the way up or down.

In this chapter and the next, I'm going to take you through the key concepts that define my Conscious Fitness approach. Each of these concepts describes a practice that helps to bring our bodies together with our minds and spirits so that our parts all work together. These practices ***create more consciousness***.

Catt's Key Concepts

Before each Set:

1. Become Present
2. Set your Intention
3. Find your Place in Space
4. Ground Yourself

Preparing to Lift:

1. Visualize the Muscle You Want to Work
2. Direct Your Energy
3. Consciously Request your Muscle to Move
4. Prepare your Muscle to Move

While this is not at all a linear process—many things happen at once—I'm going to explain each of the components in a linear order. This will help you get a sense of each. As we go through them, try to get a "feel" for how they all link together.

Also, while this list may seem lengthy, in practice it only takes a few moments. These moments will not only make your workout more efficient and productive, but also safer.

Before each Set:

1. Become Present

One day I was meeting with a client who was late. She was in such a state of stress that I could actually feel her vibrating. I just knew she wasn't ready to begin to exercise yet. So I sat her down on the piece of equipment she was going to use. I asked her to close her eyes, take a deep breath, and with my hands on her shoulders, asked her to exhale. I did a very short hypnosis on bringing her presence fully into the room, leaving her stress behind for the moment, feeling her feet on the floor, her body on the bench, and asked her to make a commitment to what was going to happen in the next 55 minutes. That commitment also involved what she wanted for herself at that particular moment. Then we were ready to go, and she was visibly different.

This happens to all of us. We live in a world of zillion distractions; we're always rushing from one place to the next, taking our upset and confusion from the last place into the next. We're seldom actually where we are; instead, we're fragmented and our energy is scattered all over the place.

When we're in that state, we're not really conscious. Therefore we tend to be careless and that makes us more prone to injury. That's reason enough to be concerned. But we also miss out on the benefits of being fully present to our surroundings and ourselves. So, my number one rule for a good workout is: Become present.

Becoming present means leaving all distractions behind. It means being fully present and being *where you are* in the moment. It also means centering yourself in your body. Often, our awareness is centered in our heads; it's removed from the center of our being, the center of our bodies. So, before you begin, you want to take a moment to move your awareness down into your body. How do you do that?

Right before you begin any exercise set, just sit quietly for a moment, and go inward. Become aware of your breath. Breathe in and out deliberately a few times. Then, begin to feel where the center of your consciousness is in that moment. If you feel it's in your head, slowly and deliberately move it down into the core of your body. Feel how that begins to shift things; notice how you begin to calm down. Notice how you become more present to your surroundings, your body, and your self.

Once you begin to get into that space, take another moment to get there as *fully* as you can. This puts you in a kind of meditative state. When you lift, it's important to give it your full *engagement*. Then there can be a conscious dedication to what's about to happen as well. So take your time to get present—and this doesn't mean you have to meditate for a long time. The more you practice, the sooner you can arrive at that state where you're ready to begin to lift consciously.

2. Set your Intentions

The next step is to set an overall intention for what you want to accomplish that day. Avoid more general intentions, intentions without specific outcomes, such as "I'm going to go through my workout." Be specific, such as: "Today I'm going to add muscle to my pecs and triceps."

When you set your intention, also include a commitment to do the best you can, with your fullest attention and engagement: "Today I'm committed to being fully present to my workout. This is important to me, and I'm going to give it my all."

Then, before each exercise, take a moment to set a very specific intention. With each muscle you plan to work that day, set the intention of *how you ultimately want that muscle to look*. You can get as specific as you want. Remember, this is all done internally; it's just for you. "I want my bicep to grow today," or "I want to create more muscle, more fitness or more strength with each rep I do."

Setting intentions just takes a moment, but it packs a great benefit. It helps bring your conscious awareness to what you're about to do. And, as we now know, there is a direct connection between our mind and body. Our thoughts can affect our muscles.

3: Find your Place in Space

The minute you step up to do an exercise, whether you're going to lie on a bench, sit on a bench, get into a machine or stand working with a free weight, it's important to **find your place in space**.

Why is this so important? I've seen people start to move and lift before they're even settled in to where they are. It means they're not really present to what they're doing. That makes for a less-than-optimal workout and, moreover, it's a recipe for injury.

How do you find your place in space? Before you **begin any exercise, especially a lift**, you want to be as **balanced** and **symmetrical** as possible. So, bring your consciousness into the specific space of the exercise you're about to do by asking yourself some questions:

- Ask yourself: Where is my body in space? Is it on the seat? On the floor?
- Then, feel into the situation. What are you feeling about where your body is and how it's positioned? *How* are you sitting? *How* are you standing? *How* are you lying?
- Assess your Balance: Are you feeling evenly balanced? If you're lying on a bench, ask yourself: Do I feel centered on the bench, or am I hanging off?
- Assess your Symmetry: We're not naturally symmetrical side-to-side; neither are our muscles. So we need to bring ourselves into symmetry. Look down. Start from the ground up. Ask yourself: Am I symmetrical, left to right? If you're standing, are your feet, are they evenly spaced? Is one foot behind the other? Are your toes pointed in or out? (Most times, they should be pointed straight ahead.)

Make adjustments to come into more balance and symmetry. This will help ensure your safety. After you've made your adjustments, lock in and then let go of thinking about it. In other words, set it and forget it.

4. Ground Yourself

When you lift, you must be stable. Stability is one of the keys to remaining injury-free. Therefore, no matter whether you're working with a machine or with free weights, you must ground yourself. By "grounding" I mean that at least one part of your body should be *solidly rooted to something stable* as you lift. Think of that as your grounding point. Another term for grounding point might be "stability point."

Oftentimes, your feet provide your primary grounding points. But your feet are not necessarily your *only* grounding points. If you're seated for the exercise, your buttocks may also provide grounding. So, your grounding points will vary and, depending upon the exercise you're doing; you may have several. Picture these as your structural foundation.

Before you start any exercise, take a moment to make sure you know what your grounding points are, and that they're stable. I call this performing a *grounding check*.

THE GROUNDING CHECK

Say you're about to do a bench press. In that exercise, your primary source of grounding will be your feet, so begin your preparation by tuning into your feet and making sure they're firmly planted on the ground in a way that gives you appropriate stability. Ask yourself: Are my feet aligned, or is one foot over here and another over there? I watch people "tap dancing" throughout sets all the time.

Then, explore your body, asking what are my other sources of grounding? Do these points also feel stable?

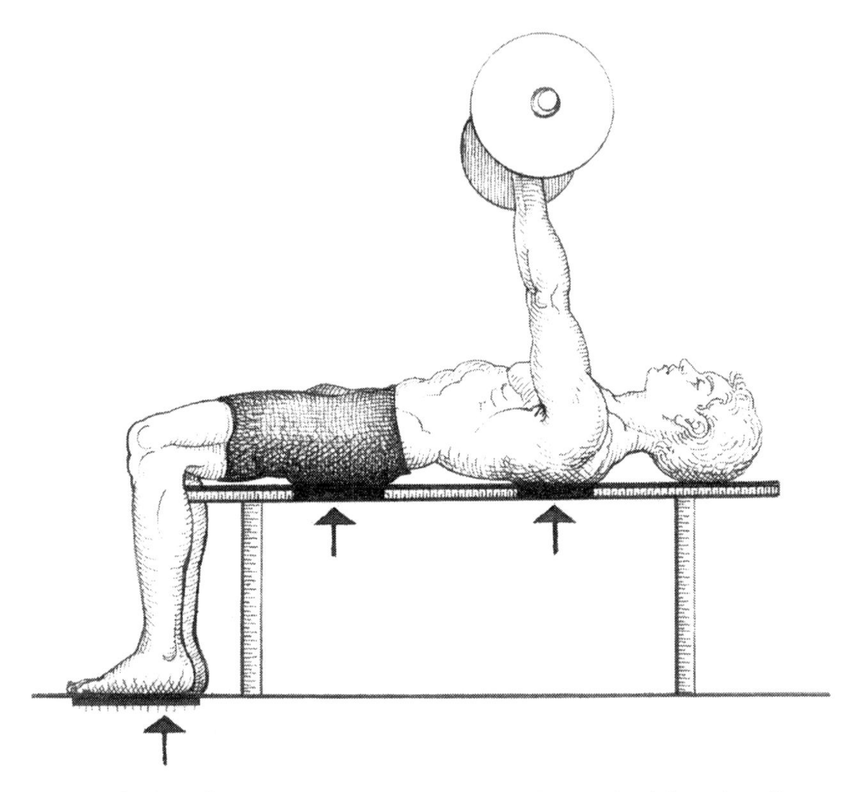

In the bench press, as you can see, your buttocks (glutes) will provide another source of stability, as will your spine and the back of your scapulas. They will each secure you to the bench, which, in turn, fixes you firmly to the ground. So, before you begin, connect with the back of your buttocks. Feel if they are firmly—and evenly—planted on the bench. If one glute is tilted left or right, it's going to change your lift motion, so adjust them to bring them into alignment.

Then, connect with your spine to make sure it's directly aligned with center of pad.

As you begin your lift, just allow the bench to support you. This may sound odd, but a lot of people don't do that. Instead of grounding into the bench, they *pull away* from it. This de-stabilizes them, which makes them more prone to injury. Continue to maintain your grounding points throughout the exercise/lift.

Whenever you proceed to push yourself into new territory, you may find yourself struggling. When you struggle, you often unconsciously and involuntarily release your grounding point(s). For example, when someone's bench-pressing a new weight for the first time and they're experiencing a little trouble, their mind will start firing, sounding an alarm and probably triggering their heart to race. Then their feet might start to "dance." They're losing their grounding. They're de-stabilizing and, again leaving themselves vulnerable to injury. They're also leaking energy, because it takes energy to move your feet, energy that should be focused on your lift. So, when that happens to you—and it will—you've got to pause and re-set both your body and your mind. Stop and take a moment for yourself. Set your grounding points again. You'll often find that re-grounding helps get you back on track, both mentally and physically.

In sum, finding your grounding points helps to stabilize you. Before you begin any exercise, perform a "grounding check." Check in with yourself to make sure you're grounded, and make any adjustments. Make sure you're stable when you make those adjustments. And remember: If you're going for your maximum weight that day, it's doubly important to be grounded, be solid, be still and not "all over the place" mentally or physically. I can't state it enough: grounding properly helps prevent injury.

THE POWER OF VISUALIZATION

Before we go further, I'd like to say a few things about visualization in general because it is such a major tool in my approach.

Visualization relates back to my core concept of hypno-fitness. *Hypnosis is essentially visualization in a relaxed state.* Our conscious mind reads words on page and goes about things logically, but the subconscious is all about imagery. If we want to unleash the power of the subconscious—and work through our limiting beliefs—visualization points the way.

In my approach, *visualization catalyzes the muscle-building process and help takes you beyond self-imposed limits.* Here's how.

5. Visualize the Muscle You Want to Work

You want to be able to *visualize* each of the muscles you want to develop. To do that well, you should first become familiar with each of your major muscles and **what it is designed to do, at its core**. That's the kind of intimate knowledge you need to build muscle most efficiently.

That's also why we took a tour of your major muscles in the chapter on the Body. After you finish reading this section, you might want to go back and review that chapter until you feel you have a felt sense of each of those muscles and how they work in your body.

Visualization is closely related to two other aspects of my approach: **directing your energy** and also what I call **conscious requesting**: *asking each muscle to do what you want it to do and grow in the way you want it to grow*. I'll talk about these next.

6. Direct your Energy

Conscious bodybuilding has many levels and layers. Here's an even deeper layer: Building muscle is an *inside job*; it's about *putting your consciousness into the muscle*—and the rest drops away.

I do that by "focusing." I deliberately ***direct my mental energy***. My mental energy isn't diffused and scattered, which is what distractions like TV and music can trigger. Instead, it's harnessed in the service of my workout.

If I have ear buds and music blasting directly into my ears, I feel that I can't "hear" my body. I might be tapping my foot to the music or thinking about the lyrics and perhaps even the memories that those lyrics bring up. Similarly, if someone, like your training partner, is talking to you, you're not focused on what you're doing, causing energy to leak away.

Focus is very important to Conscious Fitness for a variety of reasons.

First of all, a lack of focus—even a momentary distraction—can lead to injury. If you let your attention wander off, if you're talking while doing your set, the potential for damage is greatly increased. So you've got to monitor your attention and bring it back if it becomes unfocused. For example, some people choose to have a spotter urging them on loudly with "C'mon, you can do it." That's too much for me. Anything external tends to take me out of my concentration. So, if I have a spotter, I'll ask them beforehand to speak to me calmly and quietly. Of course, everyone has a different level of tolerance. Just pay attention to the kinds of things that distract you, that diminish your focus, and tone them down or move them out of your workout completely.

Secondly, it's important that you direct your **focus appropriately.** As I've said, bodybuilding is not about lifting a weight; it's about moving a muscle. We've been conditioned, though, to focus on the weight; that's where our thoughts automatically tend to go. So another aspect of focus involves changing your thought process so that your attention is on the muscle you're working, not the weight. In short, *stop thinking about lifting the weight* and *start thinking about moving the muscle.*

When you focus on moving your muscle, the weight should simply feel like it's coming along for the ride. I can't emphasize this enough. This may seem like a subtle distinction, but it's very important. Why? Because *your thoughts have power, they will affect the outcome.* Focusing on the muscle unites, integrates your mind and your body; this is a more powerful place. If you're focusing on the weight, you'll lose that advantage. It's a very different attitude. *It's mind and muscle, <u>not</u> mind and weight!* Yes, the weight's part of it, but it's not the major part of it.

Third, it's important to focus your attention on the specific muscle you want to work in the particular exercise you're doing. Do you want to make your bicep bigger, for example? If so, you need to focus on—direct your mental energy toward—that specific muscle. Thus, your focus will vary with each exercise, depending upon the muscle you intend to work.

Focus is especially important if you're doing a compound exercise, such as a squat. This is called a "compound" exercise because several joints are in action: hips, knees, and ankles. Your hip is moving and your knee is also bending; you're also balancing the bar on your back.

So you can see how it would be easy for your focus to become diffuse. When you perform a compound exercise like this, it's really important to bring you attention level up and focus your mental energy by asking yourself questions such as: *Where am I directing my mental energy? What muscles am I intending to focus on in this exercise, my glutes, or the muscles on the top of my leg? My quadriceps, or my hamstrings?*

Fourth, focus on working that muscle not only externally, but *internally* as well. As I said earlier, building muscle is an *inside job*; it's about putting your consciousness into the muscle—and the rest drops away. You want to direct your energy into the body of the muscle. My conscious approach to bodybuilding/sculpting is about **training your brain to channel energy to exactly where you want it**.

You can direct more energy into a muscle by focusing on your breath:

- As you extend, inhale *into* the meat of that muscle.
- As you contract, squeeze the breath *out* of the muscle.

7. Consciously Request the Muscle to Move

What's one of the biggest problems in relationships? We *assume* the other person knows what we want, need, or expect. We believe we shouldn't need to tell them; if they love us, they should *just know*. But most often, they don't know; they're not mind readers. But we get upset when they don't deliver. This is a set-up in which everyone loses.

In fact, most of the time even the people we're closest to don't know what we're wanting, needing, or expecting. They're so busy with their own lives, their own concerns and problems and thoughts that they can't always tune into us. And we shouldn't expect them to. There's so much static around today—so many distractions and frivolous messaging—that people's ability to tune in to what's essential is being severely disrupted. So, you're right; the potential is there, but the capacity is not well developed.

That's why it really helps to make a specific request, to ask the other person for exactly what you need, and then get their agreement. Otherwise, we're setting ourselves up for disappointment.

There's another aspect to this, too: the part about making that request in a very *conscious* way. Here's what I mean: We take responsibility for choosing what we want, and then we ask for it. I believe this practice of *conscious requesting* supports us both internally and externally. You see, if we expect the other person to read our minds, we can get really sloppy in our thinking. We don't have to get really clear within ourselves about what it is we really want. Instead, we can just get angry with the other person for not figuring it out for us. "*You should have known I really didn't want to go the party.*" "*Why did you let me buy that shirt?*" It's a way of shifting the responsibility for our lives onto others. Been there, done that! And I bet you have as well.

But when we consciously request something of others, we've taken the time and effort to first get really clear within ourselves about what we want and need. That's self-respect. Not only that, we're clear about what we're asking of the other. We've asked ourselves, on their behalf, is this reasonable and do-able? That's deeply respectful of the other person. Then, when we make the request, the other knows exactly what will please us. And they'll want to respond positively to our request because they love us and want us to have what's best for us. It's a win-win.

The same is true for your relationship with your body. If you want your body to work for you in a different way, do additional work, or to change its shape, I believe it's important to make a conscious request of your body. In fact, I'd suggest you make a conscious request of each muscle you want to work with. Include in your request all the other parts that feed and support your muscles, such as your heart, breath, blood, etc.

What goes into making a conscious request of a muscle? Take a moment to get clear about your intention, and be really specific. Do I want this muscle to change shape? Grow in size? Elongate? Become more differentiated? Develop more strength?

Then begin an internal conversation with that muscle, with the very fibers of that muscle. Ask them to do exactly what you want them to do.

When I do this, I focus my mind on the particular muscle I want to work, and I enlist my mental energy to help me move the weight. Sometimes I break it down even further. I not only ask the muscle, but I might also request my blood to flow into that muscle and oxygenate it. That's because each has its own beingness—my bicep, the blood that flows through it and even the oxygen that comes in through my lungs and flows into my blood. All those things participate in helping me lift that weight.

This idea of having a conversation may seem strange at first, but it really works. In fact, it's part of an overall strategy to become more appreciative, aware of, and intimate with your body. Again, I draw upon what I learned from my Native teachers. They talked about having conversations with all of your parts, that's what we should be doing with each muscle that we're working.

So it's important that we not only make the conscious request, but also that we show gratitude when it's granted.

8. Prepare the Muscle to Move

Before you undertake any lift, you need to **prepare the muscle**. This is really important for this reason: a muscle should *never* go directly from being slack to lifting a weight, especially in the single joint exercises. Here's why: It can most definitely lead to injury. Before a muscle can move a weight, it has to first *contract*. Think about how, if you want to make a big leap, you first pull back into a crouch. That's because you instinctively know that the crouch will give you the momentum to spring forward.

In short, you need to tense a muscle before you call upon it to perform a big task. Here's a vivid example showing why this is so important. A friend was water skiing one holiday weekend. As he was still putting his glove on, the boat's skipper turned around and asked for the nod. Not wanting to hold things up, my friend told the guy to hit it. As the boat surged forward, the line handle jumped out of my friend's hand and, in a reflex, he reached out to catch it. What happened? He tore his biceps tendon right off the bone. Why? It was because his muscle went from slack to full extension in an instant. That puts tremendous strain on a muscle. Normally, when you're properly prepared for the boat to launch, you feel the rope start to tighten and your muscles have time to make the adjustment. They tense up.

The need to tense your muscle first, before extending, is not obvious to most, unfortunately, because they've not been taught how to work with their muscles. Their focus has solely been on lifting the weight. But again, with my approach, we're *not* lifting weights, we're *moving muscle*—and we happen to be dangling weights off that movement. That's very different.

Therefore, I see lifting as a three-step progression:

1. Slack muscle
2. Tense muscle
3. Lift

When I do a leg press or squat, for example, I consciously contract first and tense the muscle before I pick up the weight. I stand under the weight, even to take it off the rack and put all my weight against it. I tighten and then lift up. I do it this way so that my muscle has a chance to register the weight.

Although I've explained visualization, directing energy, conscious requesting and preparing the muscle to move as separate steps, in reality they all blend together. Together they prepare you to lift more consciously, as we'll discuss in the next chapter.

10. Conscious Fitness Step-by-Step

LIFTING CONSCIOUSLY

IN THIS CHAPTER, I'll teach you how to lift weight *consciously*. I'll take you step-by-step through each of these seven aspects.

The Seven Aspects of Conscious Lifting

1. Conscious Lifting: The Inner State
2. Moving a muscle from its anchor point (while applying the principle of opposition)
3. Maintaining control throughout
4. Performing "running checks"
5. Staying present and re-centering as needed
6. Building confidence in your technique through visualization, touch and feel
7. Taking a conscious approach to pain

1. Conscious Lifting: The Inner State

Our energy is usually very scattered. That's pretty much the human condition. So, before I begin a lift, I engage in a two-step process, proceeding from "focused relaxation" to "focused concentration." This process enables me to gather up my energy so that I can consciously direct it into my lift.

Once I've grounded myself to the bench/floor, etc., as we discussed in Chapter 8—so that I feel safe and stable—I close my eyes (whenever possible). It's best to close your eyes because vision is such a powerful sense. We take in ten times more information visually than aurally. When your eyes are open, you're receiving lots of information, both relevant and irrelevant, and your mind is busy sorting and filtering out all that irrelevant stimuli. Even someone just walking past will draw your attention, however fleetingly. You may not be focusing on all the information coming at you, but your mind still has to process it in order to determine what to pay attention to—and that takes mental energy.

Now think about how much more brainpower you'd have available if you closed off to all those distractions. Then, all that mental energy could be used to concentrate on the muscle you want to exercise. Therefore, if I'm in a stable position where I feel safe and comfortable, I close my eyes. (Obviously, there are times when you may not want to do this, such as when you're performing a squat.)

Once my eyes are closed, I move my consciousness into a space I call "**focused relaxation**." First I relax and let everything go. I do that by closing my eyes, and taking two or three deep breaths. As you practice this, you might find it helps if you breathe up from the ground while counting "3-2-1." Notice if your face relaxes, as that's a cue that you're relaxed.

Then, to help you gather up your energy, imagine taking in all the light in the room and compressing it into a diamond.

Once I feel I've gathered up my energy, that's a sign that I've entered that focused relaxation state. Have you ever watched a cat napping? They're incredibly relaxed, but at the same time alert to even the slightest motion. It's really quite amazing how they achieve this seemingly paradoxical state without any stress. This is akin to what I mean by a state of "focused relaxation." I'm relaxed and calm, and everything else has dropped away. My mind isn't wandering; my attention is concentrated.

From that space, I enter into an even deeper state I call "**focused concentration**." This state is the complement to focused relaxation. When I'm in focused concentration, I visualize the specific muscle (or muscle group) I want to work, and focus my mind on it. As I do that, the rest of my body fades into the background.

I then use visualization to create an image of how I want that particular muscle to look and feel as a result of this exercise. For example, if I want the middle fiber of my bicep to pop more than the rest, then I actually visualize that happening. I'll visualize a specific muscle. Then I literally start having an internal conversation with that muscle, with the fibers of that muscle, asking the muscle to do exactly what I want it to do. In this way, I enlist my mental energy to help me move the weight.

Then I begin to lift—from the anchor point within my targeted muscle. I'll explain anchor point next.

2. Moving a muscle from its anchor point while applying the principle of opposition

Remember the principle I discovered through ballet: that there is *a grounding down even as there's a lifting up, away from?* That's the principle of opposition; that's what you want to replicate.

Here's the underlying idea: Your goal in bodybuilding is to thicken your muscles. To thicken a muscle you must expand or lengthen it and then contract or shorten it through repetitive movements. (The technical terms for lengthening and shortening are "eccentric" or "concentric" movements, respectively.)

To do this most effectively, you first want to "anchor" your intended movement at a specific point within the muscle. Then you move out and away from that "anchor point." This is what creates the opposition.

The anchor point is the specific place within your muscle where you want your exercise to start and stop. Generally—but not always—your anchor point will be the thickest, reddest part of the muscle. (Remember, I am always using visualization to "see" color and shape.) Anchoring your exercise in the thickest part of the muscle—and moving from that point— helps avoid injury because you're relying on the strongest part of the muscle. If you don't take a moment to anchor your movement appropriately, you run the risk of moving from a less robust part of your musculature, such as the tendons, which are much more fragile.

Say, for example, you want to develop your pectoral muscles by doing some bench presses. First, you connect mentally with those muscles. To do that, you need to visualize them, which is why you need a good, basic understanding of your anatomy. The pectoral muscles are attached to the breastbone in the middle of your chest.

Now that you've visualized those muscles, define your anchor points. In this case, we want to imagine anchoring the movement towards the innermost attachment.

This is where you want your movement to start and end. Anchoring your movement here will keep the stress as far away from the shoulder joint as possible. It will prevent you from recruiting the tendons in the shoulder—which is important, as this can lead to injury.

Before you lift, it's a good idea to visualize how your muscle is going to move. Remember, as we learned in our story of the world champion runner, Lee Evans, seeing it first in your mind's eye can help immensely.

Let's walk through your bench press step-by-step, using the illustration below to help visualize each step in the progression.

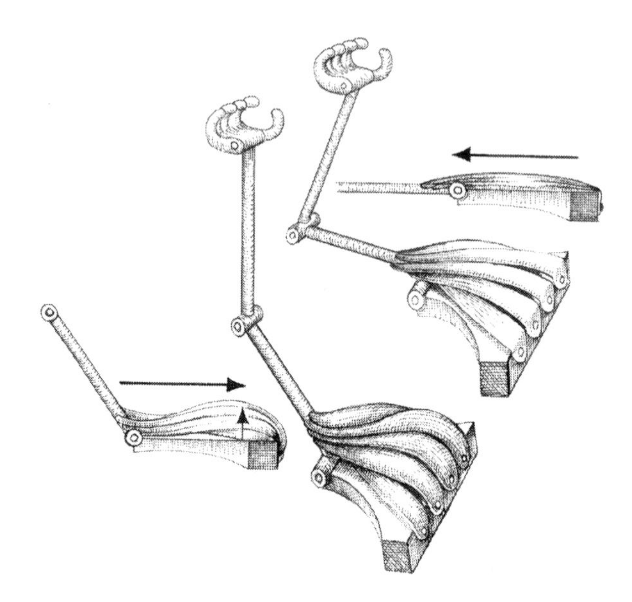

Imagine yourself getting into position. See yourself lying on your back on the bench press with the bar above you.

- Before you lift, visualize your pectoral muscles. (For the sake of simplicity, we are showing the pec attached to the simple structure of a board.)
- Then, identify your anchor points within the pecs, and focus your energy on there. (Anchor points are indicated by vertical arrow).
- Now, take hold of the weight. As you begin to bring the weight down, visualize your pectoral muscles lengthening as they move outward from the anchor points. Visualize your pecs, stretching like a rubber band from center to lateral edge. It's this kind of movement that will stretch your pecs most effectively and efficiently.
- To maximize the benefit, it's also important to elevate your chest when you do this exercise. To help with that, visualize your chest being draped over a shape resembling an inverted salad bowl. You may have to "pop" your scapulae up to create the effect of being stretched over a dome.

- When you get to the bottom of the motion, you want to re-set and contract the muscle before coming back up. Again, the movement of bringing the weight back up *begins in the anchor points*—not in your arms. Note: When you lift from your anchor point(s) in, and from the anchor point(s) out, it should feel very different from how it feels when you rely on your arms to move the weight. Can you begin to sense the distinction? If you can't yet, be patient. It takes time. It's a very difficult thing to feel, especially in the beginning. But when you get it, it is amazing!

I'm emphasizing the need to move from anchor points because this is the opposite of what we tend to do instinctively. I've observed that once there's something in our hands, such as a dumbbell weight, we tend to focus on moving the thing that's in our hands. And the way we do that, we think, is by moving our *arms*. That's how we think, but that's *not* the most efficient way to build your pecs! The most effective way to build your pectoral muscles—or any muscle—is to *anchor your movement first in the muscle*. Forget what's at the end of your arms. In fact, forget you have arms! Bring your focus to the muscle(s) you've chosen to work and visualize your corresponding anchor point(s). *Move from there*, and just let the weight come along for the ride. Imagine your pecs moving your arm up. In reality, it's a matter of sequencing. It's pecs pushing/pulling arms—not arms or hands pushing weights.

In sum, let *moving the weight be just the byproduct of the contraction of your pectoral muscles*. (In fact, if you think about it, this particular lift is a PULL, not a push. I say this because the action of contracting (shortening) the pecs forces the rigid upper arm bones Inward, and that drives the rigid lower arm bones Upward.)

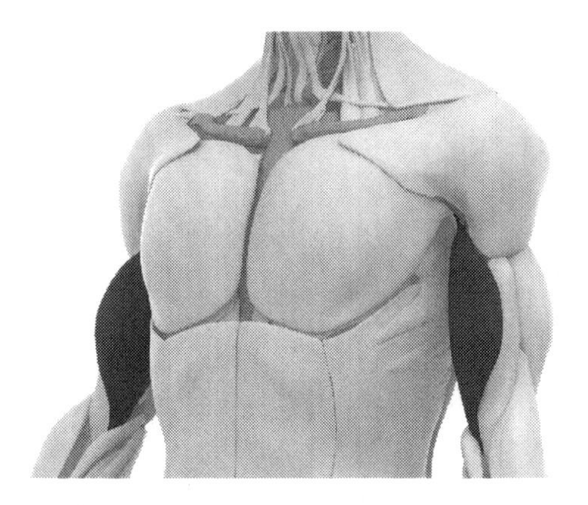

For another example, let's visualize the bicep.

As we said before, the bicep is a "two-headed muscle," meaning it's attached to the bone by two tendons (hence the term "bi"). You can see how it's split down the center. As you can also see by looking at how it's attached, the bicep's core function is to pull up your lower arm.

In general, I'll want to work my bicep from the middle, the widest, thickest part, which is the peak of the pyramid. That's my anchor point. I visualize pushing that middle peak higher when I flex. As I bring my arm down and extend the muscle, I'll consciously pull that peak down so it almost flattens. When I flex and stretch this way, I keep the tendons calm.

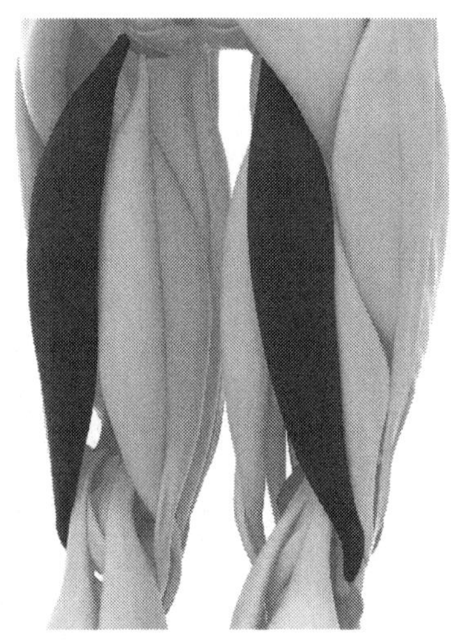

Your hamstrings function in a way similar to your biceps; one of their functions is to pull the lower extremity up.

As with the biceps, when you work your hamstrings you'll generally want to move from the thickest part.

To determine the proper anchor point for an exercise, I ask myself these important questions:

- What muscle do I intend to work? How is that muscle configured? Where is it strongest and where is it weakest?
- Which portion of my muscle do I want to *move from* so that I achieve the bodybuilding result I want?

These questions help you zero in on the anchor points. Then, as I'm lifting, I do a quick check by asking myself another guiding question: *Where am I holding the stress of this exercise?* If I'm working my biceps, all of the stress should be in the middle of biceps, not in the traps and certainly not in the elbow joint itself, as this can lead to tendonitis.

In sum, the anchor point is the place from which you extend and contract. Anchor points are a challenging concept, because they vary from muscle to muscle; they can also vary from exercise to exercise, and from intent to intent. You have to develop a feel for this, and that will only come with time—but visualization helps immensely. Again, please be patient with yourself. Keep visualizing, searching and asking yourself questions. As you keep at it, your sensitivity will evolve, I promise.

3. Maintain Control Throughout

I've seen guys taking bench press bars and literally bouncing them off their sternums, off their chests, like a springboard. That's *not* genuine weight lifting. Why? Because the goal is not to just to move the weight; it's to build muscle. To build muscle, the muscle has to be worked. If you're using momentum to get the weight up, you're not using your muscle to do it; the first six inches of the lift are just the result of spring momentum, and momentum in this case doesn't do anything for the muscle. If you're bouncing, it's just the bounce that's making the weight come up. So, if you're trying to build muscle, you're defeating your purpose.

I believe that it's much better to *control the weight at all times*. That means all the way up—*and* all the way down. As I tell myself: "Feel every quarter-inch." This is what builds muscle.

There should be constant micro-adjustments throughout the whole set to keep the weight placed in the muscle properly.

To control the weight, I attempt to take momentum out of my lifting. Now, of course, you can't take momentum totally out, but you can change how you use momentum so that you maintain more control of the weight. Here's what you need to understand to do that.

I've noticed over the years that people tend to think it's all about what they consider to be the *exertion* part of the exercise. If they're bench-pressing, they think it's only about the push against gravity; if they're doing a pull down exercise, they only focus on the concentric motion, where you contract the muscle. They tend to go *unconscious* on the eccentric motion. But that's only one half of a lift. A lift is actually a *circle* made up of two equal aspects. You need to be just as completely involved in the eccentric motion (in this case, the descent) as the concentric motion (the ascent).

When I lift, there's always tension on the muscle. From the beginning of the rep to the end, there's always tension. *Always*. No slack, even when I'm bringing the weight down. If I'm doing a pull down exercise, for example, I'll attempt to feel my back pushing the weight back up rather than letting gravity do it, as most people do. (It's more than resisting on the way up; it's actually *pushing*.) Similarly, when doing a bench press, my pec is both pushing the bar up and pulling it down.

In sum, I want power in both the eccentric and concentric motions, which means *there is no momentum*.

Learning to maintain control throughout a lift can be challenging for many people who've been lifting for a while. If you've lifted using momentum with slack at the top and bottom, you'll have this idea in your head that going down with the weight feels very different from going up. Now you have to recognize that's not so. You may have to unlearn old habits, and it can be frustrating at times. People have told me that I make five lbs. feel like a hundred. You'll find that the muscle fatigues much quicker if you don't let that tension up—and that, after all, is what we're after. Also, when you lift this way, it gets painful pretty quickly because you're not letting up. You have to learn to deal with that pain in a new way, as I'll discuss in the section ***A Conscious Approach to Pain.***

As you begin to use this technique, you'll find you can't lift as much weight as you're used to. Maintaining control throughout (and not using momentum) feels very different, and folks tell me they feel weak because they can't lift as much weight. I understand that's frustrating, because we get into this linear mindset that says "progress" is going from lifting a 25 lb. plate to a 45 lb. plate—and now they feel like they're going backwards! But life isn't linear, and linear progress is an illusion. You have to remember what your real goal is: *Is your goal just to put more weight on the bar, or to build muscle size and definition?* Besides, once you understand how to control your lift, you'll be able to slowly add weight back on. And, in time, you'll actually be able to do more because you'll have a much better understanding of what you're doing.

To help people recognize this, I slow them down so that they're lifting much more deliberately, more consciously. (It's not the "super slow" method where you count beats; I see that as a distraction.) You'll know the right pace by how you're feeling. Now, they're working their muscle not just on the uplift, but as they're going down, too.

When you lift this way, your rhythm is continuous; it isn't different when you're going down from when you're going up. It's consistent. The overall feeling is like when you're painting a wall, and you don't want brush stroke marks or splatter. You paint in a very even, controlled manner, up and then down, up and down. Visualize this right now: the brush going back and forth, not letting up. In sum:

- Don't begin to lift with a slack muscle. Contract the muscle for a full second before moving the weight.
- Maintain control throughout. Never let gravity alone take the weight down.

- Never let up on that muscle. Keep your muscle under continuous tension throughout your up-down or in-out motion.
- It should feel like painting with an even brush stroke throughout.
- Maintaining tension throughout takes momentum out of the equation. That's not easy, but has to be done for optimum results—and optimal safety.

I developed this approach because I wanted to keep myself safe from injury. Basically, I was a "scaredy Catt." I'm always amazed at how boys are so completely careless with their bodies! They don't think about injuries and, if they do get injured, they just tape themselves up and go back at it again. But then, when they're older those old injuries begin to take their toll, and the system can break down. So maybe feeling a little scared was good, especially with respect to lifting. I loved lifting heavy weights, especially in the beginning, but I was always in control. At the time I was maybe 150 lbs., benching 255. I had to ask myself, how do I bring this bar down and push it back up without hurting myself? I looked inward for the answer, and that helped me develop this technique.

Over time I discovered that it's actually more beneficial to lift this way. The reward is that I get to do this for a long, long time. I'm 58, and I've no aches and pains. I've done a lot with my body, but I've been good to it. Maintaining control really helped me, and it can help you, too. Just be patient with yourself at the beginning. Now this is not to say that controlled "burst" movements, as we do in plyometrics or as applied to power lifting, aren't valid. But know what you're supposed to feel first, and learn how to control that burst.

A NOTE ABOUT CREPITUS

Sometimes when I put my hands on someone's shoulders I feel a lot of what's called "crepitus," a crackling or creaking in the joints. In my opinion, crepitus is a sign of relying on the joint too much in an exercise. It means they're using tendon rather than muscle to move the weight. (For the exercise physiologist, a caveat: of course they're using their muscle, but too much toward the tendon "end.")

The remedy for that begins in the mind. Visualize the *muscle pushing or pulling the joint*, rather than the joint pushing or pulling the weight. In your mind's eye, see the joint itself remaining relaxed and simply articulating the motion, rather than driving it. It's a different mindset, and sometimes just by shifting their consciousness in that way, I can get people to stop creaking.

Other times, that creaking or crackling is a signal that someone isn't maintaining tension on the muscle in both the eccentric (extending) and concentric (contracting) motions. If I can get them to maintain tension in the muscle evenly on both the way up and the way down, then I can usually make the crepitus stop.

The muscle is nice thick red meaty thing. It's made for contraction. It's supposed to be doing all the "heavy lifting." So if you keep the bulk of the strain/effort on the muscle—on the anchor point of the muscle—you'll get rid of a lot of crepitus and benefit your joints as well.

4. Perform Running Checks

Remember, conscious weightlifting is about working a single, isolated muscle or muscle group while everything else in your body remains calm. If you're holding tension in any other part of your body, this will leak energy away from your efforts. So, while you're focusing intensely on a particular muscle (or group of muscles), you're simultaneously scanning up and down your body to you see if you're holding any tension elsewhere. I call this a "running check."

It sounds like a long, laborious process, but it's not. It's actually quite instantaneous once you get the hang of it.

HOW TO CHECK FOR ENERGY LEAKS

In a running check you're checking for energy leaks. To check for energy leaks, it helps to ask yourself some questions, such as: Am I *squeezing* the bar, rather than just holding it? I ask this question because we tend to leak a lot of energy into our hands. It's because we're a lot like monkeys; we're graspers. It's a natural tendency. Then, once we've grabbed onto something, our minds immediately focus on what's in our hands. And if we need to move this thing in my hand, we think we need to grab and squeeze to do so. But we don't; we merely need to *hold* it. Not only is squeezing hard on our tendons, it's also a waste of energy.

To help people break out of this habit, I tell them to *forget about what's in their hands* because it's actually irrelevant. As long as whatever they're holding—whether it's part of a machine or free weights like barbells or dumbbells—is balanced in their hands, I tell them to release their grip on it. Otherwise, their energy—both mental and physical—leaks into their hands.

Obviously, you can't have a completely open hand, but you shouldn't have a "death grip," either. When I'm working with a machine, I look for what I call the "sweet spot" in my hand, the place in my hand that I can push from without gripping at all. For example, if I'm doing a preacher curl I almost balance the bar of the machine on my palm instead of gripping it. This sets the wrist in a different way, too, so I have to keep my wrist very straight. In this way, my wrist is not flexing or extending, *i.e.*, it's not helping with the momentum. Again, it's about calming the joints that shouldn't be in action/use. In a preacher curl, for example, the wrists should be quiet.

If I'm intending to exercise my bicep, I want to feel the energy of the weight in my bicep—not in my hand. If I feel it there, it's because I'm gripping the bar too hard. I need to loosen my grip because I'm leaking energy away into my hands. Loosening my grip will shift the focus of my energy away from my hands and back to my biceps, where I want it. Here's a trick you can do yourself: When I discover someone gripping too hard, I tell him or her to imagine a ball of energy in each fist. Then I tell them to run that ball of energy from their hands back up their arms and put it in their biceps. Once they do that, I'll see them slightly open their fingers and relax their grip. Then I know they've got it.

You can be leaking energy in other places, too, so ask yourself questions like: Is my face contorted? How about my neck? Am I holding tension in it? And, because we take in so much information through our eyes, our eyes can be the source of huge energy leaks. For example, am I distracted by something I see on a nearby TV? Because we're so easily distracted visually, I often tell people to close their eyes when they exercise (but only if they're in a stable situation). We can leak energy through our ears, too. Am I distracted when I hear someone drop a weight? Is someone grunting loudly as they lift? Is my training partner keeping up an endless line of chatter? Am I too focused on the music in my headphones? Again, if you find a leak, deliberately move the energy back into the muscle you're intending to work.

You can also leak energy when you engage in any extraneous movement, such as when your feet start dancing or you're wiggling your body. These are reflexive things we often do when we're trying to lift a new weight for the first time, or trying out a new machine. And energy leaks aren't just physical; they can also be mental.

If you find an energy leak, you need to make an adjustment. You do that by first relaxing the tension. This frees up energy. Then you send that excess energy into the muscle you're focusing on. It's about taking charge of your energy and channeling that energy to where you want it. That's all part of training your brain.

Checking for leaks is relevant to any type of workout that involves muscle control, because these require such focus. If you don't shine the light of consciousness on every aspect of what you're doing, you won't be as successful. But remember, we're not talking about perfection here; these are goals. Don't ever beat yourself up. Adopt a beginner's mind. You can start over fresh every day, with every set, every rep.

5. Stay Present and Re-Center as Needed

For the first one or two reps of any exercise, you should focus on getting a feel for how to do the movement properly. Again, it's like shining a flashlight; you're looking for a certain feeling—a feeling of muscle isolation, together with mental determination and focus. Over time, it becomes an automatic thing.

Once you find what it is that gives you that feeling, it's a lockdown. Nothing moves but that muscle and what that pulls along with it.

BEGIN GENTLY, SLOWLY

Start by doing a light set of your first exercise. As an example, let's say my goal is to bench press 185 lbs. for two or three reps. I don't attempt that right away; instead, I want to work up to that. So my first set might just be the bar at 45 lbs. for 15 or 20 reps, *i.e.,* nothing strenuous. This centers me; it brings me into the present, into the room, and begins to connect me to the muscle or muscle group I intend to work. It also starts the blood flowing into the muscle, which awakens it. I follow this by doing another set with a little heavier weight. Then I'm ready to do the heavy lift. I recommend doing a warm-up like this for each body part you intend to work that day.

Warming up this way is really important. It also gives you a chance to assess how you're feeling, whether you're experiencing any joint pain, etc., and to make adjustments if you discover energy leaks. For example, I might find I'm holding tension in my trapezoids (traps), or in some other muscles. The first set is where I work on becoming aware of those things and making changes to refocus my energy.

RE-CENTER AND ADJUST

Over time, you'll develop more of an instinct about how your workout is supposed to *feel*. You'll begin to sense when it's going well. You'll also be able to sense when something isn't right. That happens to me every once in a while. I just sense that there's something "off" about my technique that day, and I can feel myself getting sloppy.

It's important to pay attention to these signs. The cause could be physical or mental. As you push yourself into new territory, you might be struggling because you find a certain lift particularly challenging. Or perhaps you've had a particularly stressful day, and you catch yourself not being able to focus.

When that feeling comes, I don't just push on with sloppy technique. Instead, I come down into whatever the stretch position is for that exercise, without putting the weight down. That means I'm not stopping the exercise; I'm pausing within it. Then I take a moment to get my body back into proper position. I make sure I'm properly grounded. Then, I just breathe and wait for new information to show up; I wait for my body to communicate with me, to tell me what I need to know.

It's in those moments that I often get a deeper level of insight. I'll see, for example, that I've had a rough day and that I'm holding that tension somewhere in my body. Maybe my neck is tense, or my jaw is tight, and this tension is preventing me from being truly present to my workout. Sometimes, it's just my mind going crazy, wanting me to stop.

I might hang out in the stretch position for ten seconds or so while I mentally re-group. Then, once I've re-centered myself, I'll return to the exercise. I'll try to eke out maybe two more reps in a controlled manner.

Taking a moment to do this when you find yourself struggling sends a message to your over-active mind. It says, "I don't quit just because you're uncomfortable. I'm committed to this exercise and I'm going to find a way to stay with it by listening to my body." In this way, you begin to train your mind to quiet down. This is like building muscle, too: the muscle of mental discipline. Your mind will get the message that you want it to work from a different place, not a place of disorganization and fear or anxiety, but from a place of clarity and calm. It's almost like training a puppy; you have to be consistent. Over time, as you practice this step, you'll notice a difference. In that way, it's like a spiritual practice (a moving meditation).

6. Build Confidence in your Technique through Visualization, Touch and Feel

You can use visualization during an exercise to help you with muscle isolation. Here's an example: The equipment frames in my gym are all bright red, and all the plates are dull grey steel. I designed it that way so folks can play off that to develop their own imagery. If someone's doing a bicep curl, for example, I tell him or her to visualize the thickest part of the bicep as glowing a bright, burning red, like a barbecue coal, the same color as the equipment frame. Then, with every repetition, I suggest they attempt to mentally see their bicep glowing brighter and brighter, as if every squeeze is like blowing on an ember. Meantime, visualize the rest of the body and cool it down to the color of that cold, grey steel; make it really still. I find that this kind of visualization helps people to isolate the bicep. It also reinforces the core concept of opposition.

You can also learn to use visualization to help you master the technique of a particular exercise. I'm fortunate in that I can visualize easily. Because I'm so familiar with my musculature, I can close my eyes and, metaphorically, peel off my skin and watch my body move. **I also see muscle** movement in geometric **shapes**. For example, when I flex a bicep, I see a pyramid.

I use that gift for visualization to help me see how well an exercise is working and to detect when folks are missing the mark with their exercise. I can see that when folks are thinking too much about the bar in their hands, for example, they come down wrong, and I can use this

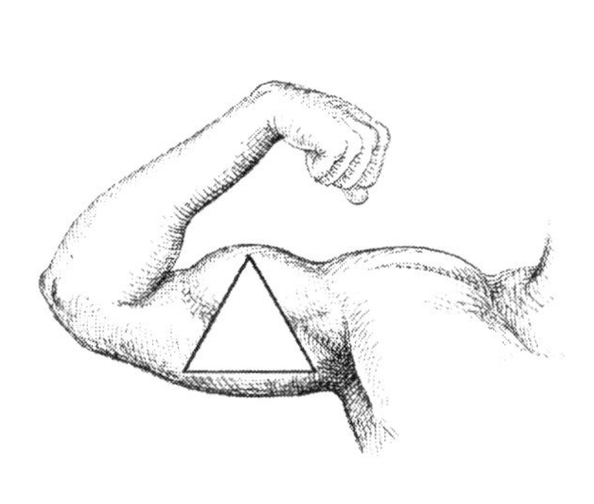
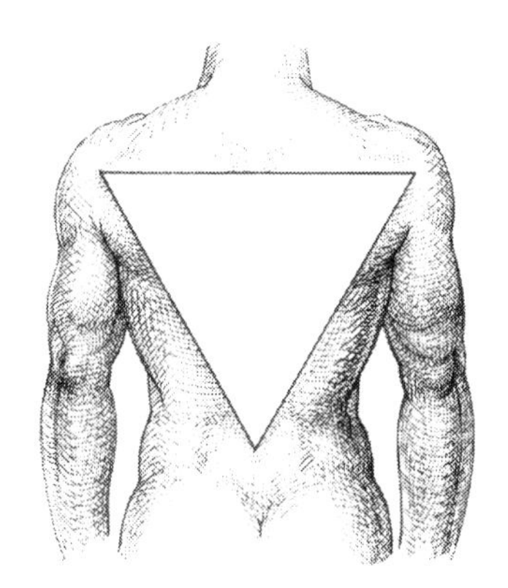

gift help people make adjustments. There are all these places where the joints have to open in order to perform the exercise properly, for maximum benefit, and I can use visualization to evaluate that.

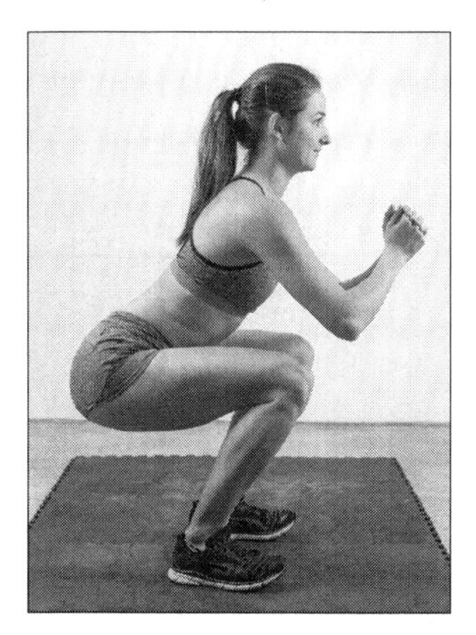

For example, a proper squat involves the torso leaning a bit forward with the hips back. Your femur is underneath the torso, and your calves also come back a bit. It's like a "Z" formation. It's a really structured exercise. When done properly, you can see that structure at work, supporting you. For example, as you come down into the squat, I see your hips, knees, ankles, and lower back as circles. As you're moving down, I see each of those circles rotate downward. As these circles rotate down, they pull your tailbone towards the ground. Then as you rise back up, the circles rotate in reverse.

The distinctions I'm teaching are subtle and may seem even impossible to grasp at first. That's one of the reasons why I find visualization so helpful. I also find that visualization is inherently personal: Different imagery works for different people. Find your own imagery, unique to you.

Along with encouraging the use of visualization, I use touch a lot to help me guide people. I might have folks put their hands on their muscle to help them feel the difference between stretching and contracting—and help them develop a tactile sense of those concepts. I may have them place their hand on my bicep so they can feel—and internalize—the difference between how they're currently pulling and the way they should pull. I encourage you to use your sense of touch to help you develop your body awareness. If you stay with it, you will begin to *feel* the difference. When a client finally sees or feels what I'm seeing or feeling, that's a magical moment.

7. Taking a Conscious Approach to Pain

Sometimes, lifting involves discomfort or a small level of pain. That's the nature of strength training. Building muscle requires that you push the muscle beyond its perceived limitations. This is what "encourages" a muscle to build—and it necessitates a certain amount of "manageable" pain.

Pain and discomfort are a part of fitness, just as they're a part of life. While many traditional cultures accepted that and prepared their members for it through initiation rituals and other ceremonies, like the Sun Dance, our culture is quite pain-avoidant. We seem to believe that pain can be avoided altogether—and that it's OK to mask it with drugs.

Conversely, there's also a "macho" attitude that says to ignore pain and push through it, even though that might result in serious injury. These are two extremes, and both are prevalent in our culture.

Because we tend to have this very confused view of pain, I'd like to share with you what I've learned about it.

WHAT IS PAIN?

At its core, pain is nothing more than *feedback*. It's an informational flow, the body's way of communicating to you. Therefore, it's also a teacher, in a sense. Most of us probably had the experience of touching a hot surface or getting too near to a flame when we were kids. That experience of pain taught us a valuable lesson about how to navigate the world. But that doesn't mean that any sense of pain automatically means "Stop!" or "Don't do that!" Pain is just pain, a tool, a form of feedback. It's how we read and respond to pain that's important.

Because pain is the body's natural feedback mechanism, we have to be able to feel it. In general, we don't want to diminish our ability to feel what our bodies are trying to tell us. Therefore, I'm not a believer in getting cortisone shots or using other kinds of numbing agents to dull pain, unless absolutely necessary. I'm not saying things like anti-inflammatory medications are inherently bad. I'm saying that pain is a feedback mechanism and that allowing ourselves to feel it can help prevent damage.

It may seem paradoxical, but pain (*i.e.,* feedback) is your friend because, if it's the right kind of pain, it's signaling you that what you're doing is exactly right; your exercise is accomplishing what you intended.

Back in the 1980s, a bodybuilder friend of mine, Mike Dayton, was pretty famous. You might see ads featuring him in the backs of comic books saying "Discover the Power of Chi." Mike would regale the public with feats of strength like tearing a phone book in half lengthwise or bending a quarter. Once, he held back a dragster for a second and a half on *Wide World of Sports*. "It's not strength that does it," he'd say. "It's being able to tolerate the pain long enough to accomplish what you've set out to do."

That, in a nutshell, is the challenge.

As I've explained previously, building muscle up requires first breaking muscle down. That's where pain comes in. Your muscles respond to being broken down by, in effect, saying: "Whoa! This is a degree of stress I'm not ready for, so I'll have to make myself stronger and bigger to handle it." In short, muscle responds to a challenge by "wanting" to grow. And it will, if you don't stop the process prematurely by bailing out.

Simultaneously, your muscle is sending you a feedback signal, in the form of pain, to tell you the process is happening. That's a good thing. But when you get that pain signal, your mind might interpret it as your muscle screaming, "Quit!" That's when you can feel yourself wanting to escape. It's your mind resisting pain. In your resistance to pain you might get sloppy in your technique or stop altogether.

But here's the next layer.

There are degrees of breaking a muscle down. A competitive bodybuilder, for example, will deliberately put so much stress on a particular muscle that the muscle just won't work any more. We call that point **muscle failure**. Whenever we get near that point of muscle failure, we can be in a chaotic state because our mind is virtually screaming at us to stop. But we don't. We learn not to run from the pain, but to go *into the pain*, into it, into it. And yet—here's the paradox—at the same time, we also *detach* from the pain because we don't want to relate to it so much that it makes us stop.

You see, there is a difference between *true muscle failure* and a *failure of the mind*. In the heat of the moment, it can be difficult to tell the difference, but learning the distinction is what turns us into champions. When a bodybuilder masters this—and it takes a while to do so—there are almost no limits to what he/she can do with his/her body.[52] Acquiring this capacity requires a special kind of consciousness, one in which you accept the input of both your body and mind, but you transcend it. Perhaps one way to describe that is to say that the spirit of bodybuilding takes over. You surrender to something larger than yourself, while at the same time continuing to be present and mindful because you never want to go overboard. You want to consciously manage the process because you want to stay safe and avoid injury.

Now this probably doesn't sound very attractive to the layman, but that's because I'm describing the extreme end of it. A layperson shouldn't take things this far. However, when you're exercising properly, you *do* want to bump into some discomfort because that's the feedback that tells you the exercise is working, that you're beginning to break down muscle to build it back up more strongly. When you feel that, that's *good pain*. (Note: What I'm calling "good pain" is not sharp, injury causing or chronic, but more of a burning discomfort—. Good pain is useful and controllable and not an indication that you're abusing your muscle.)

If you resist that pain and stop, then you won't push the muscle to that point where it begins to break down and build up; you'll break the chain. But if you can hold steady when that pain hits—even for just a fraction of a second—you can reap the rewards of a highly efficient bodybuilding process while also being safe from injury.

As a competitive bodybuilder, I learned how to apply the principles of hypnosis to help me stay with the pain even when both my mind and body were screaming to quit. I couldn't stay in that place indefinitely, of course, but I could for short bursts of time, enough to accomplish my goals. In learning to stay there, I discovered a place beyond time, and a deeper level of awareness that told me how to push myself safely. This practice helped me achieve a sense of mastery over my life. You can, too, through the technique of focused relaxation/concentration.

Here's how focused relaxation/concentration can make a difference. When you're relaxed in this way you can *allow* a certain amount of appropriate pain to be there without reacting. When you're in that state, you can just *notice* the pain; just observe it, without attaching to it or needing to do anything about it for a time—just enough time—to enable you to strengthen that muscle.

When you feel that discomfort, then you actually learn to rest in it. Yes, your body is signaling you and that will trigger your mind to tell you to leave—but you don't. That's key to Conscious Fitness. It's about corralling that pain and enveloping it with awareness. You have an acute awareness of what's happening, but there's also what I'd call a detachment of judgment. You observe, but detach. Observe, but detach. Admittedly, it's a paradox. It's like finding the calm in the eye of the storm and just staying with it. There's this quiet little place where you not only find a sense of calmness and detachment, but you also connect with the pain at the same time.

One of the techniques I use to help me detach and cope with pain involves moving my eyes rapidly from left to right. This is a variation of what's now known as Eye Movement Desensitization and Reprocessing, or EMDR. Research into treatments for post-traumatic stress seems to indicate that side-to-side eye movements can lessen the effect of distress and improve our ability to cope.[53] I didn't know about EMDR at the time; I just discovered the technique by tuning into my body; my body led me to it. I have confidence that similar things will happen for you, too, as you become more attuned to your body and its wisdom: you'll be led organically to what your body needs just as I have been.

When you deal with pain in this very conscious way, you don't have the option of running away. The part of you that wants to go away is the part that judges the pain as being something bad. But it's not; it's *just pain*. Observe it; hold it. Eventually you get to the point where you can say, "OK, so it's pain. So what?"

If you've ever practiced yoga (which I recommend), you have some idea of what I mean. You'll be in a pose that calls for stretching and you'll reach point where it feels like your muscle can't stretch any more and then, usually just when you've given up, you find a deeper place in your pose. Your muscle releases, and then it can stretch just a little more. When you experience that, it's just amazing!

The inner state you reach with yoga is similar to the state of mind I'm talking about in Conscious Fitness. It's about you commanding the muscle vs. the muscle commanding you. In that way, it's like taming something within you. The weirdest thing is looking for that pain, searching for it and finding it, and then staying with it while not attaching any negative judgment to it. So it's there, you can feel it--even see it in your mind's eye. Then you take any emotion that's attached to it—and you calm it down. Just calm it down. As my yoga teacher, Lisa, would say, "Suffering is optional."

It's being in the paradox of connecting with "pain" while simultaneously ignoring it that takes you into the "zone." And it makes you tougher in so many ways. That gives you a tremendous amount of control.

DISTINGUISHING TYPES OF PAIN

I'll push through pain; all bodybuilders learn to do this. But that said, not all pain is the same. Some pain is "bad," meaning it's a signal that you should stop what you're doing immediately. Some pain, however, is "good." It's signaling that you are absolutely doing the right thing. You need to be able to distinguish between the two, which requires a certain intimacy with your body. You have to know which pain is OK to push through, and which isn't. To do that, you have become attuned to your body. Let's consider an example.

I once overheard a gym member say that his back was "on fire" after doing a certain kind of leg workout. His words got my attention right away. I knew that wasn't a good sign, so I asked: What kind of pain is it? Is it muscular? He was a very muscular guy but, as is common, he was also very out of touch with his own body, so he couldn't tell.

In asking a few more questions, I learned that he was doing heavy Smith-machine squats. I kept probing and discovered that a year before, he'd had a motorcycle accident. I suspected a connection. But, he protested, "When I do leg presses, there's no pain." "Well, of course," I said, "There's no compression of your spine in that exercise. That's very different from having a heavily loaded bar on your shoulders."

No matter how strong you are, if you've got that heavy weight on your shoulders, your spine is going to compress (versus when you're lying down and pushing with your legs). I asked some more questions and found out that, after the accident, they x-rayed his shoulder, but never his spine. I told him to go to chiropractor and get x-rays of his back because he may have slightly ruptured a disc. If so, when he puts weight on his spine and it compresses, he might be squishing that disc that's already ruptured out a little bit, and maybe he's feeling pain because he's getting a little tap of bone-on-bone. As it turned out, I was correct. But because it didn't hurt when he was doing a leg press, he kept pushing through the other as well.

If someone's lower back hurts, there are some questions I can ask to help determine what's going on, such as: Does it feel like it's muscular? Are you getting pain shooting down your leg? Is the pain spread across the entire low back? Is it on one side? Depending upon the level of pain they're feeling, I'll refer them to someone who can help.

Some pain, as I've said, is good in that it's signaling that you're on the right track and should continue. This is particularly true of the pain involved in the breaking down of scar tissue. Here's why.

Under normal circumstances, the muscle fibers lie in uniform, linear order; they're sheathed, and they slide across one another as you move. If you look at the pecs on an anatomy chart, you'll see how the muscle fibers all go in one direction. When you tear the muscle, however, the repair process doesn't move along those same, smooth lines. Instead, it proceeds in a crosshatch fashion—with the repair tissue a more fibrous type—resulting in something like a patch that goes *across* the tear. That's what scar tissue is. Essentially, once the scar forms, you've got extra tissue in the area, positioned differently than before. Plus, the scar tissue isn't as lithe as the original. This combination creates restriction, and your muscles can't move as smoothly or well.

Let me give you a specific example. A close personal friend can't bend or straighten either of his arms fully. His range of motion is quite restricted because he tore both his biceps and now the scar tissue that formed is preventing him from fully straightening or bending his arms. Ironically, though he suffered trauma to both arms at different times, he doesn't even remember what happened to one of them. That's typical of a lot of guys, I find. They get injured, and the first thing they say to themselves is, "It's not gonna stop me." It's brave, but it's also a kind of denial; they don't want to know that they've sustained an injury. So they won't get it looked at by a medical professional, and they won't do therapy to make sure it's healing appropriately. The next thing they know, they can't do the things they used to—like straighten their arms—and they don't know why.

To complete the healing process, *you've got to break down that scar tissue*. This is a step that people often skip. When scar tissue has formed, it's necessary to do the work to break up that cross-hatching so those muscles can slide again, giving you back your normal range of motion, or pretty close to it. The way you break those down and release those restrictions is through manipulation. A good masseuse can help with this—and the right kinds of exercises are essential. These will involve some discomfort, even pain—but it's "good pain," pain that tells you you're effectively breaking up the scar tissue. (I have such a practitioner. And though I tease her about the level of pain she can induce, I couldn't imagine not having her in my corner!)

Once you start working with your body a lot, you can tell whether the problem is with a muscle, tendon, or ligament. I know whether I'm in danger of straining or tearing one or the other, or if there's a vertebra out of place. I can even tell you what therapy I need. But that's over years of training.

To know the difference between good and bad pain will take time; you need to become attuned to your body. As you progress in your practice of Conscious Fitness, you'll develop your ability to discern. You'll be able to tell if it's the right type of pain occurring in the right spot in the specific muscle you're targeting. But as you start out, I recommend familiarizing yourself with the feel of "muscle burn." Then, in the meantime, if you sense something's not good, that something may rip or tear, back off quickly. If you feel pain, check in with a trainer. Ask people who can help. Do this immediately. *With any type of injury, the longer you wait, the more the muscle tissue around it tightens (and loosens in other places)*. In short, the pathology begins to cascade down in a kind of domino effect, and it can spread quickly. So it's important to isolate it as soon as possible.

11. Workout Wisdom

WHEN YOU FIRST START TO WORK OUT, you might be shown a "routine," a series of exercises to do in a certain order, over and over again. I don't recommend getting into a routine. The only "routine" I want involves you walking through the gym door regularly. Here's why.

Whenever we have a routine we have a tendency to go on "autopilot," where we're not being present with what we're doing. Although we're used to them because we've been conditioned by a mass-produced, Industrial Age culture, rote, repetitive routines shut down our minds and dull our spirits. And as we've established, if your mind is absent, your workout will not be as effective as it could be—*because your mind, body and spirit need and want to work together.* That integration brings the best benefits.

Secondly, I believe that variation is much more beneficial than a "routine." On the physical level, variation is very important because your muscles can actually get lazy if you do the same thing every time, even if you're exercising regularly. The reason is that muscles adapt quickly. Once you get into routine, if you just keep repeating it—which is the very nature of "routine"—your muscles adapt to it. This actually fails to maximize your capacity for growth.

I believe you have to keep your muscles guessing! Changing things up is what leads to muscle development. If you vary what you do, your muscles have to pay attention; they have to adjust to each new thing, and that strengthens them. It's about keeping it fresh so the muscle never knows what's coming.[54]

Remember **Paul Bunyan and the Blue Ox**? In the beginning, both Paul Bunyan and Babe, the blue ox, were small. Paul would carry the little ox on his shoulders every day. But every day the ox got a little heavier. Paul continued to carry it and, as he did, he got bigger and bigger in order to be able to handle the heavier load. That's the story you want to keep in mind. The more stresses you put on your body, the more it has to adapt to those stresses. That's why if you do the same thing every day, in the same order, with the same number of repetitions, same number of sets, your body will say, essentially, "Oh, I'm so used to that. I don't need to do anything different. Ho hum." And your fitness will plateau.

Variation is also good for the mind and spirit. Thinking up new variations keeps our mind engaged and active; our spirit loves creativity and the opportunity to express its uniqueness in the world. I believe we're at our best when we're challenging ourselves and pushing into new territory.

In sum, that's why I don't recommend routines. Instead, I want to teach you the underlying principles of weightlifting so that you have the tools to design your own unique workouts. An added benefit is that, no matter what gym you go to, you'll be able to work with the equipment that's available. And if you go to a busy gym, you'll be able to adapt on the fly. Some of my best workouts have been because of that!

In the process of becoming more creative with your own workout you'll become more involved. You'll start understanding what works and what doesn't *for yourself,* not because somebody else is telling you something. You'll start observing how *your* body is reacting. What works for me may not work for you—but the general principles will. Many people come into the gym and just go through the motions;

they don't know how to do anything else. I want you to get creative! I want you to have knowledge so that you can go out and create the workout that's right for you each time.

From Routine to Intuitive Training

Rather than falling into that kind of lockstep routine, I recommend that you get to the point where you're so in tune with your body that you can be *intuitive*, that you go with what you feel that day. Here's an example: One day I bench pressed 165 lbs., as I usually do, with no spotter, and then the thought came to me, "I'd really like to get to 175 today." Now, I hadn't done 175 lb. bench presses in a while, but that day I was feeling very strong; the weights felt different, light. Some days they just *do*. You don't know whether it's because of your circadian rhythm or the food you ate, the rest you got, the supplements you took, or your incredibly complex hormonal system, but something's different. Your body tells you it's ready to be pushed just a little bit further.

So I put 175 on the bar and went and got someone to spot me. There are only a few people I trust to do that because they know what they're doing.

Then I started lifting the 175. I took the bar off the rack and I came down *really slowly* because I'm checking in, checking in every micrometer. I'm coming down really slow, and I'm feeling that load so that when I get down, I'm prepared to push up. I'm not just letting that bar come down—boom! As we've discussed, there's a tendency for some people have to come down so hard they actually bounce the weight off their chests. These are the guys who will tear their pecs or have some other sort of disaster, like dumping the bar.

It was easy for me to go there that day. I went with it, because it felt right. And I knew I couldn't get hurt because I had my spotter, Chuck. Chuck recognized that I was going really slowly on first rep. He saw that I was testing my body, getting a feel for how it was going to handle the increased weight. This is a hard concept for people to get, but it's what you need to start learning.

I believe it's important to *listen to your body,* first and foremost. Go with what feels right. Because the body is not a rigid thing, it's a fluid thing. This is where intuition comes in. You work with what you have that day.

While a lot of people believe in **periodization training**, I'm not sure it's always beneficial. Periodization means you do only a specific, planned workout for a period of time. For example, you might do all high reps for perhaps three months, followed by the same period of conditioning workouts, followed by strength (power) training. When it comes to bodybuilding, however, my approach is all about *connecting in with yourself* and not doing anything mindlessly. I believe that will bring you the maximum benefit. Once you start practicing you'll realize how much more intuitive you'll become; you'll start to move through your workouts with more creativity and excitement.

Designing your Workout: 9 Keys to the Non-Routine Routine

So how do you avoid a routine? **By knowing the options for creating variation.** I never know exactly which specific exercises I'm going to do until I get to the gym. The only thing I'm sure of is that I don't want to do what I did last time. It's an inspirational and intuitive approach to working out. You can create variation in your workout by working creatively with these nine elements:

1. **Body Parts** you choose to work together
2. **Order** in which you do the exercises
3. **Equipment**
4. **The Way in Which You Achieve Muscle Failure**: Do you want to work with a heavier weight? Do more reps? Take less time between sets?

5. **Grip** you use
6. **Angle** you work from - Within any single muscle workout, there are endless possible permutations
7. **Position** or Planes – Seated, standing, lying
8. **Symmetry**
9. **Type of Exercise for each Muscle**

Let's look at each of these in turn.

1. Vary the Body Parts you Work Together

The watchword for designing a workout for yourself is this: Keep it simple. By that I mean, focus on your major muscle groups:

UPPER BODY:

- Shoulder muscles: Deltoids & Trapezius
- Chest Muscles: Pectoral group
- Abdominal Muscles/Obliques
- Back Muscles: Latissimus Dorsi, Rhomboids, Teres
- Arm muscles: Biceps Brachii and Triceps Brachii

LOWER BODY:

- Thigh muscles: Quadriceps and hamstrings
- Lower legs/Calves

Think of these muscles as the tools you're going to use to create a piece of art. In a sense, they're like unformed modeling clay. With these in mind, design your workout for the day.

In general, your goal is to exercise your entire body (all major muscle groups) at least *once* in a seven-day period. With that goal in mind, you can custom-design your work out each day by varying the muscles you plan to work out.

Here are some rules of thumb to help you design your workout:

- Work *at least two* of these muscle sets each time you work out. (Note: You could choose to do more than two, but two is a good place to start.) Tip: If one of your body parts is weaker or needs more development than others, you might want to work it first.
- Alternate working your upper and lower body as much as possible. Ideally, work upper body muscles one day, and lower body muscles the next. Doing so lets you spend more time on each area. It also makes for a less daunting workout, and gives you more time to heal in between. (Tip: If you only have, say 30 minutes to workout, just focus on *one* muscle set.)
- Again, the goal is to work through all the major muscle sets in a week.

2. Vary the Order

Routine creeps into our overall fitness regime. It's so easy to fall unconsciously into a routine, like: "Monday is my chest and triceps day, Tuesday is my back and bicep day, and Wednesday is my leg day." I often see guys in the gym who have assigned a certain day of the week to each body part and they never change that order. Their routine is so rigid that if Wednesday is their leg day and they happen to miss their Wednesday workout, they miss doing their legs entirely. They're so locked into their "routine" that this makes logical sense to them. To this I say, No! If you miss a scheduled day, just pick up where you left off the next time you work out.

So now let's talk about how to create a structure in which you can vary the order. You want to work your way through all your major muscle groups by focusing on one-two muscle groups each day. So, first, pick combinations of body parts to work together, such as chest with back and quads and hamstrings. Then, don't assign them to a specific day of the week. Instead, just give each day a number. For example:

- Workout Day 1: Upper Body: Chest and back
- Workout Day 2: Lower Body: Legs (quads and hamstrings)
- Workout Day 3: Upper Body: Arms (biceps and triceps)
- Workout Day 4: Combination Upper & Lower Body: Delts (shoulders) and calves

When you think of it this way, you won't be likely to skip working your legs if you miss the gym on Wednesday, like the guys I mentioned earlier. You'll just do your legs on Workout Day 2, whichever day of the week that turns out to be. Here's a little chart that can help you visualize what I mean:

	DAY 1	DAY 2	DAY 3	DAY 4	DAY 5
WEEK 1	Chest, then back*	Quadriceps & hamstrings	Biceps & triceps	Shoulders and calves	Day off
WEEK 2	Back, then chest*	Quads	Hamstrings and calves	Triceps and biceps	Shoulders

Then, you want to vary how you work those combinations. For example, on Day 1 of the first week I might do my chest first, followed by my back. The next time Day 1 comes around, I'll reverse it by doing back first, followed by chest. Even that simple variation mixes things up. As to lower body, I suggest starting by doing quads and hamstrings together. The next week you might do quads all by themselves one day. Then hamstrings and calves together the following day. Want to throw yourself for a loop? Do hamstrings before quads.

Any combination of exercises is OK, though I don't typically do a chest and quad workout; it's just too hard. It's all about trying to find that variety. When you change the combo, you change the flavor of the workout. I'll do these combinations for two-three months; then I'll switch it up again.

Here's another example:

	DAY 1	DAY 2	DAY 3	DAY 4	DAY 5
WEEK 1	Chest & triceps*	Quadriceps and hamstrings	Shoulders and calves	Back and biceps*	Day off
WEEK 2	Chest and biceps**	Back and triceps**	Quadriceps	Hamstrings and calves	Shoulders

Typically, you'll want to alternate working your upper body and lower body, meaning you work upper body muscles one day and lower body muscles the next. Splitting it up this way means you can afford more time to each area. It also makes for less daunting workout, and gives you time to heal in between. Tip: If you only have 30 minutes one day, just focus on one body part.

On Day 1, I'll go to, say, chest and triceps, *i.e.,* large muscle followed by small. Then, on Day 2, I'll work my legs, followed by Day 3: shoulders and calves. The next week, I'll mix it up again. There's always benefit to whatever combo you choose, but to choose wisely you also have to understand the concept of *complementary* and *antagonistic* muscles. Complementary muscles work together in a similar, or complementary manner. For example, if you do a pull-down or pull up exercise, you're using your back and upper arm muscles (biceps). These muscles are functioning in a complementary fashion. Similarly, if you're rowing, you're using your back and biceps; these, too, are complementary muscles. Your chest muscles, triceps and shoulder muscles also function in a complimentary fashion. Antagonistic muscles, on the other hand, act in an opposing manner. While one contracts, the other relaxes. For example, if I want to contract my bicep, my tricep has to relax (lengthen).

Sometimes you'll want to work antagonistic muscles together, and other times complementary; this variation changes the feel of your workout. For example, I might begin by doing antagonistic-style muscles together, such as chest and biceps. Then I'll choose to work complementary muscles together, such as back and biceps.

Thirty years ago, the general rule was to work your larger muscle groups first, *i.e.,* your chest or back before the smaller muscles of your arms. But I suggest you try working your smaller muscles, such as your biceps, first. Then work your back. This will teach you things about your body.

You'll also learn things about your body by working your shoulders first and then doing a chest workout. Your shoulders and chest are intimately connected, so after a shoulder workout, you'll find that you won't be able to push as much weight with your chest as you could before—even if I've done a really good job of taking my shoulder muscles out of your bench-press. You just can't bench-press the same amount of weight. For example, I won't be able to do 200; only 175. (That's because my shoulders are no longer helping as much as they might have if I hadn't exhausted them first. Still, I'm likely to get a great chest workout without their involvement.)

Each week you'll be doing something different, so the body doesn't catch up. I might put my shoulders in with my back day, or with my chest day, just to give it something different. When you change the combo, you change the flavor of the workout, and that's a good thing. And every one of these workouts *feels* different. It all feels different, and it keeps my muscles guessing as to what I'm going to do. After 33 years, I'm still blown away at how a bicep workout can feel so different depending upon whether I do it before or after my chest, shoulders or back.

In general, try to go through all your major muscle groups at least once a week. Some weeks it takes me four days; other weeks, it takes five. That's because my legs are "hard gainers." Everyone has a body part that's fabulously responsive, grows easily, and they like working with. But our bodies aren't the same all over. Other parts are more challenging. For me, it's my legs. So I might take two days to work the muscle groups in my legs. One day, I might spend 70 minutes working my quads all by themselves. The next day I'll focus on my hamstrings, rather than doing them as a kind of afterthought at the end of my quadriceps workout, which a lot of people tend to do. Again, working those two muscle groups separately feels totally different from working them together. Variation of this kind keeps your workout feeling fresh and new, and keeps your body guessing.

Tip: *Add rest days.* And vary when these occur as well: From, say, three days on and one day off, to four days on and one off. All variations are valid, depending.

Again, it's all about learning to understand the mechanics of your body. All these things help your body progress and grow, but they also help you learn about your body if you're truly inquisitive, which you should be. In fact every time you do a set, it should be an exploration of your body. I still do that to this day. I ask myself questions such as: What am I feeling? What do I need to move? Change? If I detect a pinch that shouldn't be there, how do I get rid of it?

Because you're so attentive to what's happening in your body, there's a lot going on; yet, at the same time, it's really meditative because you're focused on one thing: on that muscle. How do I get the most out my muscle, how do I master it?

3. Vary the Type of Equipment

Here are some possible variations in the types of equipment:

- Machine or free weight
- The angle of the bench you use (*i.e.*, flat, incline or decline)
- Dumbbell, barbell or cable or pull-up bar (for chin ups) or the floor (for pushups)

For any body part, you can use a variety of those. For example, ideally you don't want to use only machines in your workout, nor only free weights. Of course, this depends on your gym. If your gym only has machines, then work with them, but the ideal is to vary as much as you can. As I said in the section called "The Non-Routine Routine," variation is very important for keeping the body adaptive. I encourage you to learn the basics, and then be a little more adventurous, a little more creative every day. The more you challenge a muscle, the more it will adapt and change. This is what builds muscle and makes it well defined. So, you need to always be looking for a way to stretch the capacity of a muscle in new, unique ways. In sum, *bodybuilding is the process of challenging your muscles to make adaptive changes in a very specific way.* Let's look at some more ways to create variation in your workout.

4. Vary How you Achieve Muscle Failure

The goal is always to achieve muscle failure. Varying how you increase the intensity of an exercise keeps your body guessing, looking to adapt. And it keeps you tuned in, checking in with your body. This keeps you engaged on more than one level. Here are a few ways to **increase the level of intensity** in your workout:

- Add weight to bar (or machine)
- Add reps to your set
- Decrease rest period between sets or doing "supersets," *i.e.*, two different exercises in quick order
- Add sets
- Do "negatives" – By this I mean overloading your lift with more weight than you can normally manage. Before you attempt this, make sure you have a spotter! Then, take your exercise into the eccentric, very slowly. You won't be able to get the weight back up alone, but that's exactly why you have a spotter. Your spotter's going to help you because you can control a heavier weight on the way down, but you can't control it/push it back up. Then, do it again, remembering to go

very slowly on the way down. Doing this sets you up for lifting a heavier weight in the future, because your brain and mind get used to the overload. Feeling the heavy weight in your hands is good practice. It strains the muscle; it requests of the muscle to adapt to the idea of a heavier weight. Doing negatives helps you break through barriers.

- Do partial reps – By "partial rep," I mean limiting your movement as opposed to going for your full range of motion. Again, here, you want to overload the bar, but now you limit your lift. When you only do a partial rep you can move more weight than usual; this introduces another form of variation. Partial reps can also begin to get your brain as well as your body adjusted to lifting more weight without undue stress or overdoing.

Each of these will have a different feel. Use *all* of them periodically.

Here's another way you can create variation: by changing up how you work with the combination of weight and reps. There are many possible combinations for every exercise, such as:

- Higher number of reps with a lower weight, or
- Lower number of reps with a heavier weight

For example, one day you might choose to develop your chest by working a lot of weight, but doing fewer reps. Alternatively, you might want to do high rep day with a lower weight. You might even decide beforehand whether you're going to do a "high rep" or a "lower rep" day. But remember: if it doesn't feel right in the moment, adjust accordingly. Some days, your maximum strength just isn't there.

5. Varying your Grip

Another way to create variation is by varying the kind of grip you use. Depending upon the exercise, there may several different possible ways to grip the equipment. Here are a few:

- Wide grip
- Narrow grip
- Cambered (slightly angled) grip
- Reverse grip
- Single (isolated or unilateral) grip, when you're working one side at a time
- Hammer grip

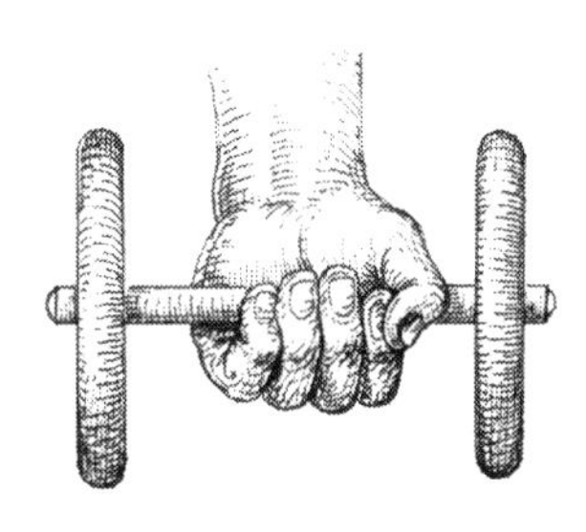

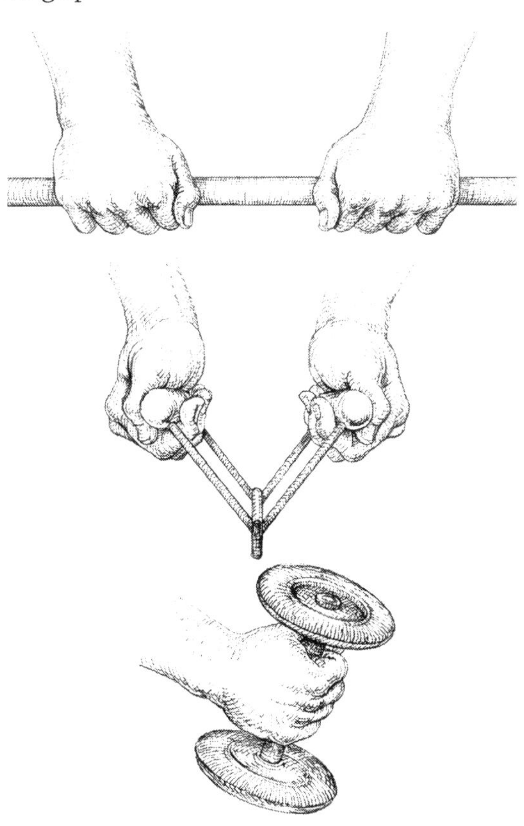

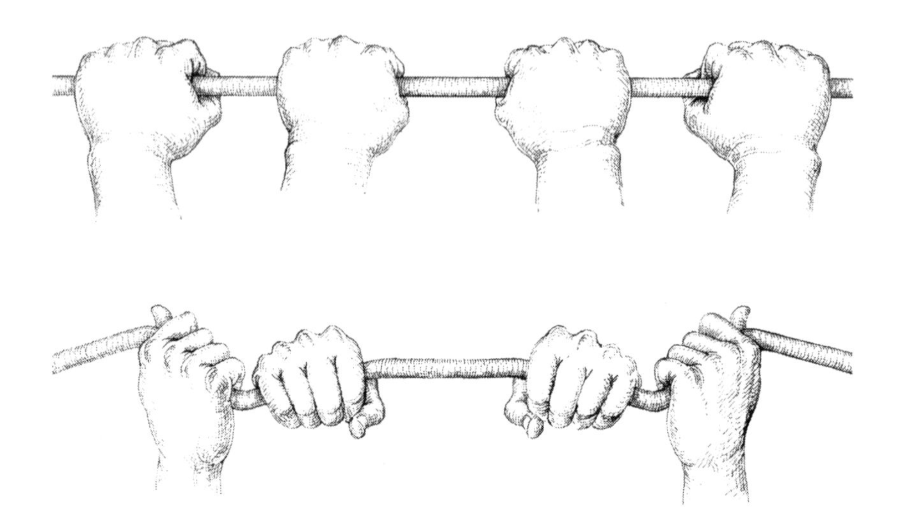

6. Varying your Position

You can also change your position to add variety. For example, here are some ways you can vary your body position:

- Lying
- Sitting
- Standing
- Incline/decline

You can also vary the position of your arms. For example, your arms can be in different positions for a bicep exercise, such as:

- Hanging straight down, parallel to my body, as in a wide grip standing barbell curl
- Behind the posterior plane of your body, such as a flat, lying dumb bell curl
- In front of your frontal plane, such as any kind of preacher curl

For lower body exercises, you can also vary the position of your legs and feet. Your feet, for example, **can be pointed straight ahead or turned out.** You might do a free bar squat in a close stance or wide stance. If you do a squat in a wide stance (where your feet are outside your hip width), then change your leg position in the next exercise you do—which could be a hack squat or perhaps a leg press. Bring your legs in such that your anklebones and the insides of your knees touch.

7. Varying the Angles

I want you to work a given muscle in as many possible angles as is reasonable in one workout. Remember Da Vinci's illustration of the Vitruvian Man?

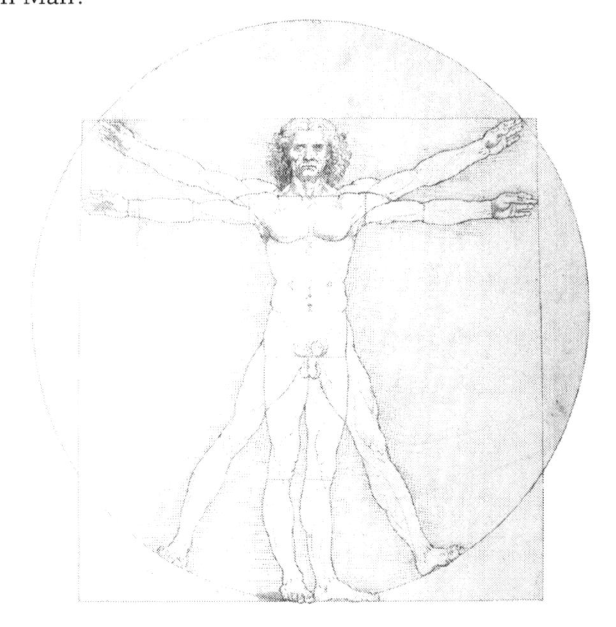

It's the perfect illustration of what I mean. It shows his arms and legs outstretched, moving at different angles around that circle. Each different angle awakens our musculature in a different way, so the more angles we employ in our exercise routines, the more fitness we evoke. (Although I'm sure that's not what DaVinci had in mind!) Now, imagine that image in 3D: we can move our arms and legs in front of or in back of our frontal plan. A workout should be as three-dimensional as possible because *we're* three-dimensional. So here's the question to ask yourself: From how many different angles can I hit a particular muscle group?

Take your back muscles for example. In one back exercise you might be *pulling* your weight *up* (*i.e.,* chin ups). In another you might be *pulling* the weight *down (i.e.,* cable pull). That's two different angles. Then you might do one *pulling back (*any kind of cable row or machine row) or *pulling from the ground up* (*i.e.,* deadlift, T-bar). These will each feel very different. It's all about keeping the muscles guessing.

8. Symmetry/Asymmetry

Another gift that ballet gave me was an embodied awareness of symmetry—or its lack—and its importance to fitness. I'm right-handed, and as I practiced ballet, I noticed that when I went to the bar to do passés on my right side, I was okay, but if I tried to do the same thing on the left, it was not so easy. I had far less control. Almost immediately, the latent scientist in me wanted to know, how do I change that?

Deborah said that I could change it by focusing on my weaker side, first in ballet class, then continuing the practice out in the "real world." If you're uncoordinated on your left side, she said, start doing everything on your left side first. For example, in my case, she suggested I put my eye make-up on my left eye first. When walking, she told me to make a point of stepping off with my left foot first. In this way, I'd begin to "awaken" my left side, which would help me create greater symmetry and balance.

There's a life lesson here: If you want to change anything in your life, the first thing you need to do is pay attention.

THE IMPORTANCE OF SYMMETRY

No one is perfectly symmetrical; that's just how our muscles are. Because all of us are asymmetrical, we all have a weaker side.

Take the time to notice your own unique relationship to symmetry. Look at your shoulders, for example. Are they level, or is one side higher? Always strive for balance between your two sides. Check in with your body. Are you feeling one side more?

Why is developing more symmetry so important? For balance and strength. In competitive bodybuilding, the judges specifically evaluate you on the basis of symmetry. That makes sense, because if you can train your less dominant side to be stronger, to take more weight, you're going to be stronger overall. You'll also be more balanced and coordinated.

Becoming more symmetrical is also good training for the brain. Working with your less dominant side helps train the brain to pay attention to what you're doing. It develops your ability to concentrate and feel your body.

Therefore, you'll want to make sure that you're including in each workout at least *one exercise per body part* that involves independent motion from each side. This could be moving dumbbells, cables or using a machine or doing lunges—any exercise where you can use one side of your body at a time. For example, say you're on a bicep curl machine. As you pull the bar up, you'll typically feel your right side more if you're right handed. So you have to make a concerted effort to be sure you're feeling it on your left as well.

Often, when I tell clients to do this, they'll tell me, "I can't feel my left side." That's honest; it takes practice. In response, I say, "Let's go back and do your right again. This time, close your eyes and really feel how you're managing your right side." This is a process I call *imprinting*. I want you to imprint that feeling as you work your right side: how it feels, what are you doing, where are you in space? Use all your senses to acquaint yourself with that feeling. Imprint it. Then go back to your left side and try to lay that imprint over what you're doing. Try to replicate the feeling of the right side on your left. Most likely, it won't come immediately, but it will come with time.

SYMMETRY AND GENDER

I've noticed this funny phenomenon: When it comes to working out, men and women tend to focus on different parts of their bodies. Men want to work the upper body, abs and up. Because legs are difficult to work, often painful, many men don't do them. (Sorry, guys!) Or they work them with much less intensity. As a result, some men tend to have big upper bodies and underdeveloped legs.

Women tend to do the exact opposite. They're worried about the shape of their thighs and butt, so they won't work their upper body as much. Both are ignoring something.

If you want to be truly *fit*, you want to make sure you're working the full body. The body wants this balance. In fact, *men will actually develop a bigger upper body if they also work their legs.* It's the way the body works. Plus, you have a lot of muscle in your thighs, so you get more leverage for lifting weight. Guys, if you want a bigger upper body, start working your legs. It's a well-known fact in the gym.

WORKING WITH SYMMETRY IN THE NON-ROUTINE

You can work with symmetry to create variation in your "non-routine" by utilizing iso-lateral movements along with bi-lateral movements. Here are some ideas:

- You may want to work one side and then the other. For example, you can do a leg press in a machine with one leg, and then switch. You might do a walking lunge: left/right, left/right. Or a forward lunge, alternating first one side then the other. You can also vary which side you start on.
- Leg extensions—people almost always move the weight with both legs, but no matter what, you'll probably have one leg taking over. Do one at a time and see how different it feels.
- Do a lying leg curl one at a time. Go through an entire leg workout with independent motion from each side: One-legged leg extensions, one-legged leg curl, leg press, lunges, etc. This is a very different workout from doing everything together.
- Start doing everything on your non-dominant side first. For example, if you're lifting dumbbells and your tendency is to go right, go left first.

9. Vary the Type of Exercise you do for Each Muscle

There are a myriad of exercises we could use for each muscle group, so don't get yourself locked in to repeatedly doing only one type of exercise for a certain muscle group, meaning don't restrict yourself to just doing pressing movements for your chest. Rather, you can best develop your chest by varying the type of exercise you do, such as:

1. Flat barbell bench press
2. Fly machine
3. Incline dumbbell presses
4. Push-ups

In the first exercise, you're lying flat. In the second, you're sitting upright perpendicular to floor. In the third, you're on an incline. In the fourth, you're using the floor to push yourself away from. You've also gotten the variation by going from working two sides together to working each side independently. Here are some examples of what variety in angle, equipment and symmetry might look like:

BICEPS: Machine preacher curl Standing barbell curl Incline dumbbell curl	ABS: Crunches Reverse crunches Planks
BACK: Wide-grip pull-ups, Dumbbell rows Close grip pull down	SHOULDERS/DELTOIDS: Overhead machine press Front barbell raise Dumbbell lateral fly Rear deltoid machine fly
TRICEPS: Lying tricep extension with a cambered bar Reverse grip cable pushdown, Tricep dip machine	QUADS: Leg extension: Lunge of some sort Leg presses
HAMSTRINGS: Seated hamstring curl (machine Single leg lying curl (machine) Stiff-leg deadlift	CALVES: Seated calf raise Angled standing calf raise Single calf press on leg press

Other Enhancements to your Workout

Pyramiding

Pyramiding is a framework you can use to design your whole workout. Pyramiding is a technique for gradually working to your way up to your maximum weight. It's a way of getting into heavier weights safely and to the best of your ability. It's also about feeling—checking in on yourself to see what you're going to be capable of doing that day.

I recommend **pyramiding** because just throwing your maximum weight on the bar right away generally doesn't work very well. Even a marathoner will run a couple of miles before a big race. Nothing kills your ability to lift a heavier weight like going to it too quickly. If you pick a pair of 50 lb. dumbbells off the rack as your first set, for example, your mind is likely to go, "Oh man, this is really heavy"—and you're pretty much done. But if you work up to it—which is what pyramiding is—it's less of a shock to your mind and your body. You're also being kind to your muscle by letting it get familiar with what you're asking it to do. It's about having respect for your body and muscle. Plus, it takes a while for me (and maybe a lot of people) to get into the flow. I tend to get better as a workout goes along. If that's true for you, too, pay attention to that. So, why not ease into the heavier weight as your workout goes along?

To pyramid, start with a lighter weight and do a (relatively) high number of reps. Then you keep adding weight while reducing the number of reps, as necessary. You finish off by doing a few reps with the heaviest weight you want to lift.

If you pyramid up, you might also pyramid down. Pyramiding down involves gradually taking weight off the bar as you increase the number of reps. We call these "drop-sets."

Say I'm doing an exercise like squats, and I want to see if I can get to a weight I haven't lifted for a while: 200 lbs. I figure I might get only 1-2 reps with that weight. Here's the pyramid approach I'll take 99% of the time:

- First, I'll do a set of 15, lifting just the bar. That's to get the blood flowing.
- I might sit at the lowest point for a few seconds creating the "template" for the feeling; the fullest range of motion.
- Next I'll move to a fairly light weight, say 95 lbs., and do another 15 reps. That won't kill me either.
- Then I'll put 135 on the bar. And while I probably can do 15 relatively easy reps, I'll only do 10.
- After that, I'll put 155 on the bar and do 6 reps. I could probably push to 12, but I'll just do 6 because I don't want to exhaust the muscle just yet.
- I'll put on 185 lbs. and feel the situation out. Again, I'm testing. If I find I'm going "balls to the wall" to lift 185 for 4reps, that tells me that I probably won't have enough energy in my muscles to get to 200 today. So then I'll stop and begin to pyramid down.
- If, however, I can do 6 easy reps at 185, and it still feels good, then I'll put 15 more lbs. on the bar and try for my goal of 200 lbs.
- I'll more than likely be able to do 2-4 reps at 200 lbs. And again, I'm testing. I could stop there. But if it still feels good, I might do another set with that weight.
- Then I'll pyramid down for one or two more sets to ensure I get some decent mid-range reps in.

This is just an example. Conversely, I might start doing squats and decide that my body doesn't like doing them at all that day. So, I'll stay lighter for three sets and move on. This flexibility serves to make a more interesting connection with your workout and helps you practice tuning in to your body.

Stretching

Can you have both strength and flexibility? Absolutely, yes. Many people think you have to sacrifice one for the other, but you don't. That's where stretching comes in.

HOW I DISCOVERED STRETCHING

When I was still involved in competitive bodybuilding, I had an intuitive sense that I should work with the fascia. The word *fascia* refers to the structure of fibrous, connective tissue that surrounds our muscles, muscle groups, blood vessels, and even our nerves. Fascia binds some of these together while permitting others to slide over each other. Think of it as shrink-wrap for the muscles. Once we paid little attention to fascia but we're now learning how important fascia is to the integrity of the human body.

My goal at that time was to make my muscles larger, all over. I started thinking if the **fascia** that wraps around all the muscles of the body, like Saran Wrap™ surrounding a sandwich. Could that be limiting the size of my muscle? It seemed logical that it could.

So, I thought, if I can open the fascia up by stretching it, while simultaneously elongating the muscle, then it would allow for the growth of more muscle mass. It was just a matter of physics.

At the time, I didn't believe science would have backed up this idea, but that's not unusual. Bodybuilders have often felt the medical community was behind in acknowledging things we already knew intuitively about the human body. We were living laboratories because we were experimenting on ourselves all the time.

When you've been a bodybuilder at the level I've been, it's not unusual to find yourself disagreeing with some of the things the medical community says because you've seen the exact opposite happen. For example, you hear so much about horrors and dangers of steroids, but then you know guys personally who take massive doses with no medical supervision. You see that steriod use might cause some issues, but how harmful are they really? Is it blown out of proportion compared to other things? If I swallow a bottle of aspirin, for example, I'm dead. By that standard, steroids are much less potentially harmful. Then there's the fact that, today, prescription drugs have surpassed car accidents as a cause of death. So how do these things really compare? I'm not making light of steroid use, but when you see these disconnects and distortions, you realize the medical community has some blinders. It starts you looking inward, to yourself, for the information about how to grow, make things change, adapt, etc. You still take information in from the outside, but you start looking within for veracity.

In addition, all new knowledge starts with an intuition, a discovery, a step into the unknown, doesn't it? It comes from noticing something and allowing your imagination to take you into new territory. EMDR, the stress-reducing eye movement technique mentioned earlier, was discovered quite by accident. While out walking one day, Dr. Francine Shapiro noticed that the distressed feelings she was experiencing abated significantly as she stopped to observe the movements of ducks on a pond. She realized that, as a result of those rapid eye movements, she felt calmer and more relaxed.[55]

Everything new starts with a willingness to push the boundaries of what we think we already know.

So, because I had this hypothesis about fascia, I started doing stretches in between every set. If I was working on my biceps that day, I was also stretching biceps. In between reps, I'd stretch as my rest. That's how I let my heart rate come down to recover for the next set.

I would stretch my muscle hard—not to the point of tearing, but to slight discomfort. And while I was sitting in that slight discomfort I'd be thinking, where can I give a little more? Can I stretch more? Where can I let go? Even to this day, I'll be stretching and thinking I'm really stretching and then I'll go: Oh, wait a minute. How much more is there? What do I need to let go of?

Stretching became important to me as a way of maintaining my focus. I find stretching really helps people new to working out especially, to locate their muscles and feel them without the distraction of moving weight. Then they can take that knowledge into their set.

For me, stretching was a kind of *active rest*. Instead of just resting and waiting for my body to be ready for the next set, I could use stretching to keep that muscle engaged and my mind connected.

Another benefit of stretching was that I became both strong *and* flexible. When I went to my first yoga class, the participants were amazed at my flexibility. They saw muscle and thought "muscle bound," but that's another myth! Keeping your muscle pliable is a major deal. Also, if you stretch your body, you make your mind more flexible as well. That's the mind-body connection again. So when we face challenges, as we often do in life, that ask us to stretch, we can respond more easily because we're flexible in both body and mind. The template's already there.

Stretching Pointers:

1. **Stretch every muscle group.**
2. **Stretch the muscle you are working in between every set.** If you're doing bicep exercises, for example, then in between every set you stretch your biceps—rather than just resting. The benefit of **stretching** the muscle you just worked in between sets is that it really teaches you where that muscle is.
3. **Duration:** Stretch each side for about 20 seconds in between every set.
4. **Don't "fight" your stretch.** Many people who go into a stretch fight their stretch, meaning you'll go into a stretch, feel some resistance, and then not allow that muscle to go further. When you go into a stretch, you're asking the muscle to open. In response, you naturally tighten. Then what? Your mind thinks, "I'm going to stretch, but it's not giving, so I've got to force it!"

No! It's actually the opposite. It's about realizing that you need to let go and "blossom" into the stretch. It's all about letting go.

When I'm stretching, doing yoga for example, the cool thing is every day I feel something new. When I do a yoga stretch, if the instructor keeps me there long enough, I quiet my mind. I start doing those running checks—then I think, Omigod, I'm holding in my left buttock, for example. The moment I realize that, all of a sudden, I get another inch in the stretch. I go somewhere I've never been before, and it's wonderful!

There are, of course, naysayers, people who now say stretching is not good. But I've been doing it for 33 years, and I'm here to say, Yes it is! And if you truly listen to your body, you'll intuitively know how much is too much for you. (A caveat: HYPERMOBILITY in the joints can masquerade as FLEXIBILITY in the muscle. Unless you can really feel the difference, find a trainer to teach you how to stretch muscles, not ligaments.)

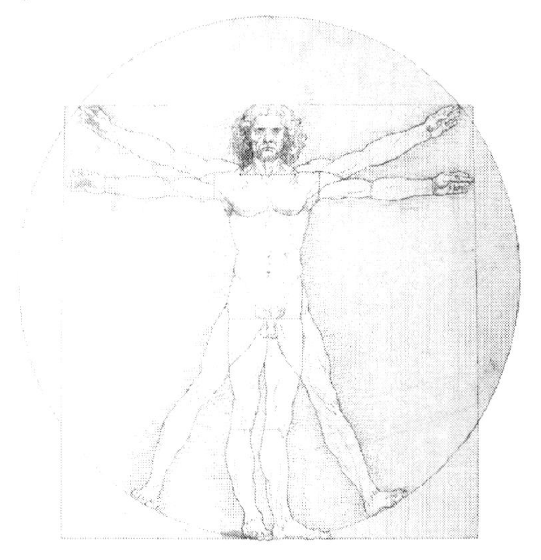

Range of Motion

I believe that exercising for the fullest range of motion is imperative. What do I mean by this? It takes us back to the DaVinci drawing of the Vitruvian Man. Note how the figure depicts full extension of both arms and legs.

This is the ideal to which we want to aspire: **full extension and full contraction in the widest possible range of angles.** Again, this is the ideal.

Why is full range of motion important? It not only strengthens your entire body, but it's the best way to prevent injury. I say this because *injury is most likely happen when the body is unexpectedly moved in a way it hasn't before.* So, if you've extended as far as you can, your body is less likely to be uncharted territory. Your body knows the terrain, and so does your mind. Because you've set up neurological pathways, your brain's used to going there. Therefore, a sudden, unusual movement will be less likely to create a great shock to the system.

I must also tell you that not everyone agrees with me on this. The National Academy of Sports Medicine doesn't. They don't want any movements involving more than a 90-degree angle. They're trying to err on side of caution, to set standards to help avoid injury altogether. I understand this—but it's not real life. What if you're a football player and you haven't trained at those lower ranges? I think it makes you vulnerable. If you accidentally get pushed beyond a 90-degree angle during a play, and you haven't stretched/strengthened in that range, you're more likely to get injured. Badly. That's not logical to me. So I say that the "no angle less than 90-degrees" rule doesn't hold, unless you're dealing with an existing injury that you have to work around. I'll talk more about how to work with injury later, in the Appendix.

Summary

With these **principles** in mind, you can build your workout. The point is, no one should become bored, neither in body nor mind. Develop a big enough repertoire so that never happens. As you become more experienced, you'll discover there are so many more possibilities for creating more variety in your workouts.

12. Conscious Eating:
A LOVE STORY

MY CHILDHOOD may have been difficult in some ways, but with regard to food, it was idyllic. I grew up surrounded by an abundance of fresh, nutritious, whole foods. The part of California where I spent most of my childhood was fertile and sun-kissed. For a kid, it was a paradise. We had peach and apricot trees in our back yard, and we'd just pick fruit off the tree and eat it whenever we were hungry. Or we'd ride our horses around the countryside filled with orchards of pomegranate trees and orange groves. There were wild loquats. Do most kids even know what these are? In the summertime the temperature was often between 110-112 degrees, and things were ripening all around you—you could smell them. And when you picked fruit from a tree and ate it, it was warm from the sun. To this day, I don't like cold fruit because I remember the pleasure of eating a sun-warmed peach. We'd feast on those and on ripe apricots. They were so perfume-y and redolent and soft. Today I can't find apricots like that to save my life.

Today, many kids are removed from the sources of their food, but it was just the opposite for me. I learned to forage for it. I plucked it from a tree or pulled it out of the ground. With my father, I picked olives from trees, gathered wild mustard greens and cactus fruit. And with my mother, I gathered wild dandelions. There were almond trees in our neighbors' yard. With his permission, we'd gather them, cracking open the raw almonds to find this nugget in a green pod. I wonder if people really know about almonds any more. (Of course, they know about "almonds," but do they know how they grow? What they look like on the tree?) We also had wild asparagus growing in our backyard. It was never enough to make a meal, so we'd just eat it raw out of the soil.

The food I grew up with was a combination of cultivated and wild. This was partially driven by economics—our family didn't have much money—but also by my mother's thoughtfulness. We grew a garden every year, and had several fruit trees as well. Most of our fruits and vegetables and herbs came from there: tomatoes, peppers, zucchini, basil, parsley and oregano. I remember watching her canning tomatoes and kneading flour for our homemade bread. In the winter, we'd go out as a family to forage for wild mushrooms. We'd return with whole grocery bags full, and she'd parboil them and freeze them to use as ingredients for her mouth-watering pasta sauces.

Food was a community affair. My mother knew all the people around who grew or raised fresh food. She knew someone who kept bees and she'd bring home jars of honey, drawn from five-gallon, stainless steel canisters in her barn. The air in the barn was heavy with the sweet smell of honey, and I remember being fascinated by the golden ribbons running down the side of the glass as she poured this beautiful amber liquid into a jar. It, too, had the most amazing smell.

Another friend raised chickens, so she'd get the freshest possible eggs from them. There is nothing like a really fresh egg! Someone else she knew had a cow. She'd come home with milk in her own container, a gallon jar with a screw-on lid. She'd skim the cream off and we'd take turns shaking it until it turned into butter. Then we'd have pure, nonfat milk. I remember having cereal in the morning that consisted of hard wheat berries that she'd cook until they'd broken open. Then she'd put on honey and milk. (She used to call it "ladybugs" because of the way it looked.) It was a glorious way to start the day.

I feel very blessed that I grew up with the connection to food that I had. We weren't wealthy, but I had a sense of abundance around food. Out of a sense of taste that was somewhat innate to their Sicilian culture, along with economic necessity, they created an ethos around food that was close to perfect. My mother, in particular, set an example. She was a bit of a magician, I think, an alchemist of sorts, who practiced the beautiful, seductive art of food preparation in such a way that I was enchanted and hooked for life. She never saw it that way; she said she cooked peasant food. I could just feel how whole the food was.

My mother also believed that every physical ailment had a natural cure. If my nose began to itch with the beginnings of an allergy, my mom would give me local honeycomb to chew. And there were other cures as well. There was red wine vinegar for swimmer's ear—you could hear it sizzle when she put the drops in—and garlic for everything. As a kid, I don't remember ever going to a doctor or pediatrician. I have such a good immune system now, and I believe she's the reason why.

When I was growing up, fish was cheap and beef was expensive, so we didn't eat a lot of red meat. In fact, we ate only small amounts of protein. Mostly, our diet consisted of homemade red sauces and pasta, cheap cuts of meat (leaner, not much marbling fat), liver, and soups made from garden-grown vegetables. We didn't have fancy desserts, either. Instead, my mother would peel us an orange or apple, with maybe some freshly cracked almonds or walnuts. Today, this way of eating is known as the "Mediterranean Diet." It's a diet that's rich in fruits, vegetables, nuts, legumes and fish. It relies on olive oil and actually encourages the moderate consumption of red wine. It's been scientifically proven to reduce the likelihood of a heart attack, according to a monumental study published in the New England Journal of Medicine.[56]

This way of eating continued even when we moved to Tennessee. We incorporated the local fare into our repertoire. For example, we learned what poke sallet was.

It was simple living by today's standards, but it was the most wonderful way to grow up. My best memories of childhood always revolve around food and food preparation. All those experiences connected me to food and gave me a sense of appreciation for where it comes from and how beautiful it can be.

I'm grateful for this amazing connection to food, because how you eat when you're a kid sets your metabolism for life. That's why it's so heartbreaking to see a five-year-old who's already 20 pounds overweight. They're going to have to fight to keep extra weight off for the rest of their lives. If we care about our kids, if we care about ourselves, we've got to change the way we relate to food.

Eating Ourselves to Death

For most of history, hunger was the central survival issue, so locating food was a central preoccupation. Back in our prehistory, we had to hunt and forage for food, often risking life and limb. We were hunter-gatherers to begin with, roaming in search of sustenance. Then we discovered sedentary agriculture and began to settle down to tend our crops or herds. We toiled on small farms, at the mercy of the weather, diseases or the landlord.

We were insecure about having enough food, and it's as if our bodies retain that historical memory of food scarcity, and it still drives us in many ways.

Once, it took a great deal of energy and hard work to produce one K-calorie. Now, largely due to industrial farming, pesticides, ambitious chemical tinkering and genetic engineering, the amount of energy needed to get that one K-calorie has dropped precipitously. Food—or food-like substances—are plentiful, at least for many of us in the U.S. We don't have to work hard for our food; in fact, now many of us have to work hard to avoid over-eating.

Our society, in particular, has seen a very significant change in food production. It's happened so fast—largely since World War II with the rise of industrial food production. Calories are plentiful, but our mindsets and habits haven't caught up.

Because it took so much effort to get food to consumers, being heavy was once a sign of affluence. Now it's the exact opposite; it's the thinner people who are admired. After all, they've withstood all the temptations of cheap food and excessive eating, so they must be superior!

Today, the daily caloric intake in the U.S. exceeds our needs. Depending upon their level of activity, men need between 2-3,000 calories per day and women between 1,600-2400—but we're eating much more. According to the U.S. Department of Agriculture, Americans consumed 523 more calories *per day* in 2003 than we did in 1970. If we eat 500 more calories a day than what we actually need to fuel and maintain our bodies, we consume *3,500 additional calories per week*. Eating at that rate, we gain *one pound per week*, or 52 pounds in a year. This helps explain why the USDA reports that 75% of men and 64% of American women are overweight or obese.[57]

The great tragedy is that a higher caloric intake doesn't necessarily mean we're getting the nutrition we need. This is because so many of those calories are "empty." In fact, if we eat the typical American diet, we're getting plenty of calories, but not much nutrition value in terms of vitamins or nutrients—with tragic results for both individuals and our society at large.

What is the "Typical American Diet?" Here's what one writer says: "Unfortunately, Americans have some of the worst diets in the world, and everyone else knows it. With the average American consuming 24 lbs. of artificial sweeteners, 29 lbs. of French fries, and over 600 lbs. of dairy per year, Americans are in a state of crisis."[54] Slowly but surely, the typical American diet has come to be laden with *sugar, salt, and fat*, a deadly combination. Of those *extra* 532 calories the USDA tells us Americans consumed each day in 2003, 292 were from added fats, oils, sugars and sweeteners.[59]

And what's so wrong with sugar? The consumption of sugar can cause a cascade of chemicals. The sensation is a quick high followed by a quick crash. We've all felt it. The candy bar lures us with its promise of a fast energy hit when, in reality, we need to eat things that burn more slowly and keep us going throughout the day. But sugar is so addictive that I consider it a drug.

In addition, we're in a cultural swirl that keeps telling us that "more" is "better." If a little is good, we think, more *must be* better, particularly where food is concerned. The bigger the portion for the dollar, the better the value, right? In fact, *restaurant portion sizes have quadrupled since the 1950s.* According to the Center for Disease Control and Prevention, hamburger and French fry meals have tripled in size over the decades, and the serving size of soda is six times larger today.[60] Could this be at least part of the reason for the ballooning obesity epidemic?

It gets even worse. This massive increase in portion sizes is accompanied by highly processed foods involving the heavy use of questionable ingredients. The majority of processed or "fast" food today contains a plethora of controversial, possibly toxic, substances such as MSG, aspartame, neotame, dimethylpolysiloxane, and sodium phosphate, to name a few. Even something as simple as "strawberry flavor" consists of nearly 50 different chemicals. Ingredients like these are used throughout the mainstream food supply."[61]

And just what are these additives? MSG, for example, has no nutritional value; it's there because it has an addictive quality. "It's nicotine for food," wrote one critic.[62] Another additive, dimethylpolysiloxane is "an anti-foaming agent" used in Silly Putty.[63] Neotame and aspartame are artificial sweeteners considered by some to be neurotoxic (*i.e.*, harmful to our nervous systems) and immunotoxic (compromising to our immune systems).[64]

As a nation, we just don't eat right. We're getting tons of calories now, but we're not getting the proper nutrition for each calorie we consume. This phenomenon is so pervasive that it's been given a name: "stuffed and starved" by food activist Raj Patel.[65] Worse, the American diet of highly processed food laced with added fats and sugars is responsible for the epidemic of chronic diseases that threatens to bankrupt our healthcare system. When we look at how much illness and disease is the result of a poor diet—in the richest country on Earth—we should be shocked. The CDC estimates that three quarters of U.S. healthcare spending goes to treat chronic diseases, most of which are preventable and linked to diet: heart disease, stroke, type 2 diabetes, and at least a third of all cancers.[66]

No one should be a Type 2 diabetic, as it's caused by poor diet, but diabetes is an epidemic in the United States right now, spreading like wildfire with no end in sight, particularly amongst children. Nearly 19 million Americans have been diagnosed with diabetes and another seven million are living with it but unaware they have it. Scariest of all are the 79 million people who are headed down the road toward being diabetic (what's called "pre-diabetic").[67] It's estimated that diabetes treatment costs alone run to $116 billion/year.[68]

The Centers for Disease Control and Prevention also estimates that 80% of heart disease and stroke, 80% of type 2 diabetes and 40% of cancer could be prevented if only Americans were to do three things–*stop smoking, start eating healthy, and get in shape.*[69]

The Politics of Food

Change begins with awareness, so let's continue to explore the big picture for a moment. As one writer states, "The health care crisis probably cannot be addressed without addressing the catastrophe of the American diet, and that diet is the direct (even if unintended) result of the way that our agriculture and food industries have been organized."[70]

In brief, the majority of the food industry is not on our side. As the author of *Salt Sugar Fat: How the Food Giants Hooked Us* puts it: "The public and the food companies have known for decades now...that sugary, salty, fatty foods are not good for us in the quantities that we consume them. So why are the diabetes and obesity and hypertension numbers still spiraling out of control? It's not just a matter of poor willpower on the part of the consumer and a give-the-people-what-they-want attitude on the part of the food manufacturers. What I found, over four years of research and reporting, was *a conscious effort*—taking place in labs and marketing meetings and grocery-store aisles—*to get people hooked on foods that are convenient and inexpensive.*" [71] And, I would add, addictive.

Yes, many of us are addicted to bad food and, while we must each take responsibility for our own health, many food manufacturers have been—and still are—acting like the "pusher man," their staff scientists working away in their chemistry labs finding ways to get and keep us hooked on substances that detract from both our individual health and the wellbeing of our society. It's an adversarial situation. Finally, we're beginning to wake up and realize that the food industry is not that different from the tobacco industry. They're now being blamed for the problem from all sides — academia, the Centers for Disease Control and Prevention, the American Heart Association and the American Cancer Society.

There's been another complication, which is that food is subject to political pressures from lobbying groups. Segments of the food industry, such as the beef industry or the Dairy Council or companies like Monsanto that are heavily invested in the genetic engineering of foods, employ very strong lobbying groups. They're able to exert such pressure that the government can be co-opted into giving us incomplete information.

Another snarl comes from the fact that—again because of strong lobbying—growers of certain crops, such as corn, wheat and soy receive government subsidies.

> Between 1995 and 2011, $18.2 billion in tax dollars subsidized four common junk food additives—corn syrup, high fructose corn syrup, corn starch, and soy oils (which are processed further into hydrogenated vegetable oils). [72]

Because corn is subsidized, it's very cheap. And because it's so cheap, high fructose corn syrup, a very sugary substance, is added to almost all processed foods to make them sweeter.[73] What that means is that our tax dollars are actually contributing to making "junk" food—*i.e.*, "food" that is both addictive and bad for us—ever cheaper, while food that is good for us, like organic fruits and vegetables, are not significantly subsidized and thus have become more expensive. According to Tracie McMillan, the author of *The American Way of Eating*, healthy food is well on its way to becoming a luxury product only few can afford.[74]

In sum, we've gone through an era that looked, from the outside, like abundance, but which actually led to negative health impacts. Along the way, we lost our way. We got seduced by fast, cheap "food" and forgot to connect with real food, slowly and lovingly prepared. Today, many of us don't have a clue about how to know if we're eating healthy food or getting the right nutrition. And we're so disconnected from the sources of our food that it's become easier and easier to confuse us. How many kids know that eggs come from chickens, or that beef comes from an animal? Many think it comes from the supermarket.

That lack of knowledge makes us vulnerable to manipulation.

Then, even if we know how to eat, it's become harder to get the proper vitamins and minerals from our food because of all the damage that's been done to ecosystems by industrial farming, which tends to disregard the need to be in harmony with nature. Crops are not rotated in a way that replenishes the soil. Farmlands suffer from topsoil depletion so manure and chemical fertilizers are over-used to "feed" the soil. Factory farms contribute to pollution. They often concentrate an unnatural number of animals in one place, which creates an unmanageable amount of waste. On a factory farm containing 35,000 hogs, for example, over four million pounds of waste are produced each week—over 200 million pounds each year. The creation of such enormous quantities of waste has a devastating effect on the surrounding air, water and soil. In addition, the overuse of machinery and irresponsible feeding practices contribute to air pollution, while chemical fertilizers and pesticides have turned agriculture into a leading source of water pollution in the United States.[75]

In short, industrial food production is in need of reform because the costs, however you measure them—economic, environmental, gastronomic or moral—are just too high.[76] But it won't happen until we stand up and demand better. For that to happen, we've got to become more knowledgeable. We've got to educate ourselves about food, about nutrition, and take back our right to nurture ourselves.

Taking Back Control

We have to begin to take back control of how we eat. That means we have to become more conscious about it.

For one, we have to respect the physical body and its requirements. If you're a parent this is particularly important. Parents need to realize the role they play in setting their child's metabolism. It starts in the womb, where the mother's diet affects the metabolism of the fetus. Then, how they feed a child sets their metabolism, not to mention gene expression, for the rest of their lives. If, as a child, your eating patterns are unhealthy, it's very difficult to reverse these later in life, especially on your own. That's one reason why, as adults, we find dieting so challenging—we're working against these very strong patterns, patterns that were set in childhood, before we were making conscious choices.

We also have to understand the nature of fat cells. If you eat too much, these cells divide and replicate, which causes you to gain weight. If you subsequently diet and become thinner, these cells don't go away; they only shrink. The truth is there's no way to get rid of fat cells; once you acquire them, they're with you forever. That means those fat cells are *always lurking in your system*, ready to be "turned on" again by over-eating. That's why the more overweight you are, the harder it is to lose that weight.

We think we can outwit those fat cells with technology, with liposuction. But the truth is that once you suction those cells out, the body then wants to replace what it lost, so it begins to reproduce those fat cells. Another technological fix is the gastric bypass whereby the intestines are shortened so that you tend to eat less. But this is a drastic measure. It sets in motion a cascade of negative health effects.

So, we've got to acknowledge this simple truth: There's no way out of eating right to support your body. That's the "bad" news. But isn't that really good news?

Eating more consciously begins with how you shop for food. How can we get more nutrition value for our food dollars? When I go to the grocery store, I don't shop from a pre-determined list. Instead, a trip to the grocery store is about feeling what kind of food my body is craving to best sustain itself. I love to handle fruits and vegetables to get a feel for whether the food I have in my hand is what I need today. It's as if these foods actually speak to me. I believe that's because fresh, natural food has a certain vital energy. We know now, through quantum physics (if not indigenous cultures), that everything is, at root, energy. Energy is alive; it needs to be in motion. When energy is moving, it has a certain vibration. If we're sensitive enough, we can sense that vibration. When we eat that food, that energy becomes part of us, and fuels us in a really beautiful way. I believe it's possible to perceive that energy, and to know if it's in tune with our body's needs. That's a very conscious way to shop for food.

I go food shopping almost every day with that in mind, looking for the freshest ingredients I can find. Even though our lives are very busy, I encourage you to do the same, as often as you can, and to practice tuning into the energy of the food itself. See if you can sense the life force energy in fresh vegetables and fruits. See what you're attracted to. The trouble is that it's hard to get that feeling from the food in many chain grocery stores. The food in many of these stores doesn't feel alive. Instead, the food's energy is so diminished that it almost feels "dead". Either it's been picked days and days ago, traveling miles and miles before it reached the store, or it's been filled with toxins—pesticides and other chemicals. Or both. Or it's not real food at all, but "pseudo-food" made mostly in laboratories where it's packed with sugar or corn syrup (a form of sugar) and sodium. And calories. Stay away from those foods (and stores) as much as you can. This will help the other parts of your life be more whole.

My Native teachers taught that there's an energetic imprint on everything. Our food picks up the energetics of everyone who was ever involved in bringing it to your plate—and, when you eat it, you take all of that energy into you.

Let's think about what that means. If you're eating in a restaurant, it means your meal has picked up the vibration of the people preparing your food. If they're feeling angry or resentful or frustrated, that vibration is part of what you're consuming. Going farther back in the food chain, think about the animal protein you eat. If those animals haven't been raised properly, if they've been given bad food or raised in abusive environments—which is very often the case today—you're consuming those negative energies. Likewise, if the animal hasn't been slaughtered humanely, you'll pick up the vibrations of their stress and fear. Likewise, packaged food picks up all the vibrations of all the people who process it, who chop it up, pack it and drive it to the place where it's frozen, packed, shipped, etc. Food that's come out of industrial farming, that's mass produced and served at a fast food restaurant will have a very different energetic imprint from food that's been grown organically, tended by a committed farmer, bought at a farmers' market, and lovingly prepared by a chef who's put a lot of thought into the meal, honoring of the ingredients and choosing those seasonally, etc. If we tune in, we'll notice that those two meals will have a very different feel. Served in a restaurant, those kinds of meals are expensive but, thankfully, we can do this at home. When I eat at home, even if I make only the simplest meal, my body is happier than if I had gone out to eat.

I used to get takeout food all the time when working a lot, but I just didn't feel good about it. I'd rather be responsible for my own ingredients and energy. And I'm a busy person. If I can cook at home, you can, too. So here's one more definitive statement: *If you want to be fit, you have to learn to cook. Period.* Now, I don't mean that you have to become a gourmet cook or that you have to master a lot of complicated recipes—not at all. In fact, I believe that we've made cooking seem too complex by making chefs into celebrities. I think that contributes to making the rest of us feel inadequate; we're daunted by the idea that we can't do it, or that it will take hours. Actually it should only take you about 20 minutes to turn out a healthy meal, to eat simple and fresh food on a daily basis.

One way we can begin to take back our power is by learning to cook—in our own homes. Learn to make a handful of good, nourishing, simple meals without following a recipe. Recipes are like training wheels; they work well to get you going, but you shouldn't feel like you need them forever. If you're just following a recipe, you'll go a little unconscious; you won't feel the food. For example, if I give you a great recipe for Caprese salad and you try to make it in the dead of winter, it's not going to taste very good. The tomatoes aren't farm fresh; the basil hasn't ripened in the sun. Develop enough skill in the kitchen so that you can buy what's fresh that day, and improvise.

On the way home from work, for example, I'll stop at the store and, while I'm there, I'll check in with my body: What kind of meal would best support it today? If I've worked out hard, I might opt for grass fed beef, but only occasionally. Most times I'll go for fresh fish, organic chicken, or pasta. If I'm really pressed for time, I pre-prepare in my head before going shopping. Then, I pick up the freshest vegetable, and a protein I can prepare easily. Fish is the fastest, easiest to cook.

Say, for example, I pick up a great piece of rock cod. It's easy to put a great meal together around that. I'll season it with salt and pepper and sauté it in a pan with some olive oil while I'm steaming a vegetable or making salad and cooking a red potato in the microwave. In five minutes, it's done. I'll just squeeze some fresh lemon on the fish and enjoy a beautiful, simple meal. When you do this, you realize that simple stuff just makes you feel better. We don't need to put melted cheese or butter all over everything. I love a good new potato with just salt and pepper. They're so creamy; you don't need butter. You have to break out of the cycle of wanting to taste butter, but if you begin to eat more nutritionally, you'll soon find that you can't stand bad food anymore—and you'll see weight come off.

Speaking of weight, it's ironic, but many overweight people are actually not eating enough. Again, it's because we're so distant from our bodies. We need to put a certain amount of energy into our bodies in order to ignite the process of burning energy. In short, you can't succeed by starving yourself; you need to consume calories in order to burn calories. We also need to understand that thousands of years of conditioning have programmed our bodies to react to perceived starvation; if our body "fears" not getting enough energy, it will store energy in the form of fat. To keep that mechanism from taking over, it's better to keep the fuel supply steady and moderate. Eat smaller meals throughout the day rather than starving yourself in between larger meals.

Each of us needs a fundamental understanding of how our body's metabolism works. Our bodies are basically energy systems; we need to consume a certain amount of energy, in the form of calories, just to keep our brains and all our other systems functioning. That's the baseline number of calories we need. If we eat more calories than that in a day, we need to keep our "engine" running hotter so that it can consume those calories without turning them into fat. That means we need to exercise in order to burn those calories. To manage our metabolism properly we need to have some sense of what we're taking in and using every day so we can keep those two things in a state of healthy balance. And to do that, we need at least a rudimentary knowledge of what your food consists of. Many people don't know what a calorie is or whether any given food contains protein, carbohydrates or fat. This is a basic understanding we all need to have. Then, you need to find your rhythms with respect to what you take in and what you expend.

If you're in a very bad place regarding food, I suggest starting with small steps. Just change how you eat one day of the week. On Tuesdays, eat healthy food. Now you're 1/7 better than you were! Then, when you're ready, add a second day. Maybe commit to only two healthy meals that day. Don't be too ambitious because you'll set yourself up to fail. The same holds with exercise. Start with a commitment to work out twice a week. Do that for 21 days. If, during that time, you really feel like going to gym a third day in the week, great! That's gravy. But if you miss a day, don't give up on the whole week. Set yourself on a schedule you can live with. If you do 50% better on your fitness and 50% better on your food, you're 100% better!

The Spirit of Food

I remember being in a class in which my Native teachers asked us to imagine being in a place where we were totally calm. Once we'd all created that imaginary sanctuary, they asked us to come back into the room. Then they passed around a plate filled with those big red globe grapes. They asked us to pick two, and to hold one in each hand. Then they asked us to pop one into mouths and experience the taste. I remember it tasting good, but not great.

Next, they had us close our eyes and go back to that quiet place we'd created and meditate on whatever we felt or saw there, just sitting with that. Once we were fully in that experience they asked us to pop the other grape into our mouth. I'm a skeptic, but the juices from that second grape were so alive that they almost leapt out of my mouth! I was astonished at the difference.

That little experiment showed me how the state of one's mind affects what we experience. It also showed me how important it is calm your mind, to be in a state of openness and receptivity when we eat. Otherwise, we miss out on the experience of the food. It's not a big step from that to considering how our busy, often harried lives affect our relationship with food. When we eat on the go, in an anxious or unconscious state of mind, we won't really connect with our food. It won't nourish us the way it would if we ate calmly, in a serene state. I saw how this could definitely contribute to over-eating, because we're constantly seeking after that experience of intense pleasure, but we can never have it because we're not in a state where we can receive it. It's a vicious cycle, a descending spiral of seeking but never attaining satisfaction because of the circumstances of our lives.

I think that part of the reason that many of us have a problem controlling our appetites is because we feel empty inside. It's like there's a huge hole and we're trying to fill it with food. We feel so empty that we keep eating even when we're physically full, packing ourselves with way too much food at a sitting. Why is that?

The "hole" is, I believe, representative of our separation from spirit, a separation from God, from the Divine. There's a disconnection from what animates us and makes us human. For many of us, organized religion hasn't provided what we need. The Judeo-Christian story of humans being cast out of the Garden of Eden reinforces that sense of separation. We feel like God or Spirit is so far removed, up high somewhere, beyond our reach. So we give up. We're drawn to secular things, to "lower" things. Remember our discussion of the chakra system? When we don't feel rooted in our sense of being and our right to be alive, we seek ways to fill that void. Sex, drugs and rock 'n roll—and food, to coin a phrase. We can overindulge in them because we're trying to fill that empty hole. "Pseudo-foods," those that comprise empty calories without real nutritional value, are designed precisely for that purpose. They're meant to feed a "constant craving" that is never satisfied and leads to even more abuse.

We need to shift our relationship to food so that we don't see it as just a way to plug that void inside, but as something sacred in itself. Food provides us with energy. It contributes to our life force. We have to reinvent our understanding of the purpose of eating. It's to feed the body, to give it what it needs for its best functioning. It's not about sublimating our emotional problems, and it's not just about satisfying hunger. Hunger, after all, is merely nature's way of getting us to take in the nutrients we need. So satisfying hunger is not the goal; nourishing your body is.

I believe that if we make a connection to the spirit of things around us, we won't abuse them. If we connect to the spirit of water, we won't want to pollute it. If we make connection to the spirit of our food, we won't abuse it either. So I work on deepening my awareness of how much I have to be thankful for and how I mustn't take it for granted. Every night, I take a few moments to thank Spirit (or whatever you want to call that Energy is that is the Source of everything) for another day, and for all the people and things that support me every day. Every evening, I take a few moments to say "Thank you for getting me through another day, for getting me home, for a roof over my head, for a safe place to sit and offer my gratitude. Thank you for giving me food, for my health and the health of all my friends and my animals." I thank Mother Earth and the farmers and all the forces, human and non-human, who brought this food to my plate because I recognize that, without them, I'm not eating. I thank every animal and plant that gave its life energy to support me and my life. I say thank you to each for its energy, which is now flowing through me.

It's a quick prayer—if you want to call it that. It's an acknowledgement of my *relationship* to all other beings and of how dependent I am upon other energies for my existence. I try to never forget that.

I believe that taking a few moments every evening to acknowledge everyone and everything that contributed to our life before we eat makes us more conscious of our food, more conscious of what we're eating and where it came from, and of its energy fueling our bodies. And if we are more conscious, our eating habits will change. Eating then becomes a kind of sacred ritual, rather than an unconscious action. In his book, *The Shaman Within: A Physicist's Guide to the Deeper Dimensions of Your Life, the Universe, and Everything*, Claude Poncelet, PhD suggests the following:

> *As you prepare to eat, with your intention, briefly connect with the spirits of the plants and animals that are about to feed you. Express your gratitude for the fact that they gave up their lives to nourish you. Express your gratitude for the fact that they have offered you the atoms and molecules of their bodies to replenish your own body. Express your gratitude for the fact that they are raising your awareness of the interconnectedness of everything. You can add that when you die, you want to offer the atoms and molecules of your body to nourish plants and animals.*[77]

Or, if all of that is too much for you, just take a few moments of gracious "noticing."

Eat the Rainbow

Earlier, we talked about everything on Earth being made up of vibrations. The scale of those vibrations in Nature is vast. It begins with sound, then climbs the vibratory scale until it reaches up and manifests as the light spectrum. Each color on the spectrum represents a particular rate of vibration.

My Native teachers taught that colors are not just beautiful; they are really important to our health and wellbeing. Our body, too, is made up of different vibrational wavelengths. When these are clear and in harmony, we feel a sense of integrity, health (*i.e.*, "wholeness") and wellbeing. But we can fall out of harmony; we can become "disintegrated" and "out of sorts." When we're in that state, a rainbow of colors has great healing potential because a rainbow is very whole in its essence. A rainbow is innately harmonious because it goes from one end of the light and energy spectrum to the other. Exposure to a rainbow of light can help clear our body of stale or otherwise unhealthy energies. They taught us an energy clearing technique called a "Rainbow Wash" where we experienced bathing in each of the colors of the light spectrum.

Just as a rainbow can cleanse our spirits, bringing all the colors of the rainbow into our bodies supports our being in a state of wholeness. When our bodies are strong and whole we're better able to withstand all the static that is constantly bombarding us from our external environment. We are energetic beings. Because our being vibrates on so many levels, we need the support of the whole spectrum of energy to sustain us. We need a variety of color in our diets because the logic of color is that each represents a different wavelength of energy. That's why I advise eating each color of the rainbow each day.

I perceived this intuitively, but it also has a scientific basis. Naturally colored foods contain what are known as *phytochemicals*, substances found in plants that have been shown to have protective or disease preventive properties. These are now becoming recognized as being so important to health that one class of phytochemical, carotenoids, are becoming known as *the seventh nutrient*, joining protein, carbohydrates, fat, vitamins and minerals (and, more recently dietary fiber) as the foundational nutrients for a healthy body.[78]

Phytochemicals give fruits and vegetables their colors. Carotenoids, for example, are plant pigments that turn on bright orange and yellow color. Good sources include carrots as well as pumpkin, sweet potatoes, squash and cantaloupe; they're also present in many green vegetables. In the body, carotenoids are converted into vitamin A and help support the function of white blood cells (healthy immune system), promote bone growth, and help to regulate cell growth and division.

Caretenoids are also powerful antioxidants that have been shown to fight some forms of cancer.[79] Antioxidants do this by neutralizing what are called "free radicals," unstable molecules that attack other molecules in the body, creating cellular damage that increases the risk of cancer and other health problems and accelerates aging. Studies show that eating foods naturally rich in antioxidants reduces the risk of cardiovascular disease as well.[80]

Eating the rainbow is an idea that works on many levels. Create more balance in your life by eating more consciously. One way to do that is to focus on bringing more (natural) color into your diet. Remember, a beige diet equals a beige life! To help you do that, I've included this chart[81] to show some of the phytochemicals contained in foods of the various colors of the rainbow, and how they help us stay healthy:

RED: Apples, cranberries, red grapes, pomegranates, raspberries, strawberries, watermelon, pink or red grapefruit, tomatoes, radishes, red peppers, red onions

Resveratrol: Neutralizes free radicals and may inhibit inflammation. Good Sources: red wine, red grapes, purple grape juice, peanuts and some berries. [82]
Lycopene: A diet rich in this may reduce the risk of prostate cancer by as much as 35 percent. Good Sources: tomatoes, watermelon, pink grapefruit, bell peppers.

ORANGE: Oranges, papaya, tangerine, carrots, pumpkin, sweet potatoes, squash, and cantaloupe

Beta-Cryptoxanthin: Plays an important role in vision and in bone and cell growth. Good Sources: Papaya, tangerines
Alpha-Carotene: Converts to vitamin A in the body; bolsters immunity. Good Sources: sweet potatoes, carrots, winter squash, cantaloupe

Hesperidin and Naringenin: These powerful flavonoids stave off inflammation and blood vessel damage caused by poor diets.

YELLOW: Apples, peaches, nectarines, mangoes, grapefruit, pineapple, yellow peppers, sweet corn, yellow tomatoes, lemons
Bromelain: This enzyme may ease indigestion and asthma. Good Source: pineapple

Bromelain: This enzyme may ease indigestion and asthma. Good Source: pineapple
Limonoids: May lower cholesterol and protect against breast, skin, and stomach cancers. Good Sources: citrus
Lutein and Zeaxanthin: These caretenoids keep eyes strong, protecting the retina and reducing the risk of cataracts and age-related macular degeneration. Good Sources: corn, leafy greens

GREEN: Apples, green grapes, kiwi fruit, honeydew melon, kiwi, avocado, broccoli, spinach, okra, artichoke, zucchini, lettuce, celery, asparagus, bok choy, mesclun, turnip greens, kale, watercress, collard greens. Dark green vegetables are nature's food powerhouse.

Chlorophyll: May decrease the risk of liver cancer. Good Sources: Present in virtually every green plant food such as watercress, leeks, arugula, parsley (even pistachios!)
Apigenin and Luteolin: Neuroprotective; may fight diseases like Alzheimer's. Good sources: Celery, parsley
Catechins: May lower LDL (bad) cholesterol. Good Source: greens
Isothiocyanates: Help purge the body of potential carcinogens. Good Sources: Kale, brussels sprouts, broccoli

BLUE/PURPLE: Raisins, blackberries, blueberries, plums, purple grapes, eggplant and purple cabbage, purple figs

Indoles: May slow the metabolism of carcinogens. Good Sources: purple cauliflower, purple cabbage

Ellagic Acid: May lessen the effect of estrogen in promoting breast-cancer cell growth. Good Sources: berries
Anthocyanins: These improve brain function and balance; may reduce the risk of cancer, stroke, and heart disease. Good Sources: red cabbage, eggplant, grapes, berries
Flavanoids: Contribute to the maintenance of proper brain function and blood flow. Good Sources: Berries, cherries, red grapes, red wine, dark chocolate, cocoa and some teas.[83]

Eat the Rainbow every day: The World Health Organization recommends that we eat at least 5 portions of fruits and vegetables daily. Fruits and vegetables are rich in minerals, vitamins and fiber and low in saturated fat. Plus, research has shown this could *reduce cancer rates by 20 percent.*[84]

Begin with your first meal of the day. Here's what I might have for breakfast: An egg-white omelet with zucchini and spinach (green). Along with that, I'll have an apple (red) or an orange. That way, I've already incorporated three fruits/vegetables, and two colors. Another day, I'll have Greek yogurt with fruit such as cherries, or some other berries (red or blue). Eating this way is an expression of artistry for me. Even when it's very simple, I can relish the colors I put on a plate or in my cart when I go grocery shopping. If you don't like the taste of vegetables—find a way to change that. Your cooking method means a lot. You have to start experimenting until you find the way that works for you.

More of Catt's Tips for Eating Consciously

- We've been convinced that convenience is more important that anything else, but it's not; it's your health that's most important.
- Many of us rebel against restrictions—is eating healthy really a restriction? Tune into how a particular food makes you feel. Does your body really want it?
- Good food is available to us, and it's truly a shame if we don't take advantage of the bounty of this Earth. Think of eating as a sensuous experience, meant to be pleasurable and nurturing.
- Learn what's in your food. Read the ingredients labels. Better yet, no labels—shop for fresh food. Acquaint yourself with where your food comes from. It comes from the Earth and our relations, the other living beings—plant and animal—that inhabit the Earth. It doesn't come from McDonald's or the freezer.
- Eat as naturally as you can. If you haven't already, start making the shift to organics. Beware of packaged foods! Not only are processed foods full of potentially harmful additives, but the packaging itself can also be harmful—as has been proven with respect to the linings in cans.[85] If possible, cut back on food that comes in boxes, bags, and cans. No artificial colors. For one week, try not to eat any "food" that is labeled at all (with anything other than price and weight).
- Go to the grocery store as often as you can. Buy food that's seasonal. This puts us in tune with the rhythms of nature. This is important because our bodies are naturally attuned to the cycles of nature. Frozen vegetables are less healthy for us than fresh. Shop for what looks good that day.
- Think balance: We need protein, carbohydrates, fats, vitamins and minerals, fiber—and phytochemicals. Alcohol in moderation; red wine. The same with dessert. Fried food? Maybe once

a week. If you eat something "bad," counter with something good, like a salad to help usher it through and clean it out.

- Think about the source—where your food comes from matters. We need healthy proteins, fats and carbohydrates. When it comes to animal proteins, it's important that this energy comes to you in a natural, sacred way. Buy only grass-fed beef, free-range chicken and wild-caught (not farm-raised) fish.
- Salt, fat, and sugar are addictive. Use them sparingly. For kids, no sugared cereals. Make bowl of "ladybugs" instead. Hard wheat berries crack open when they cook and look like ladybugs. Eat them with honey and milk—a chewy, delicious breakfast.
- We need variety. It's not good to eat the same thing, like broiled chicken and brown rice, every day. Remember, the goal is *not* an austere lifestyle, but a life that is rich and lived to the fullest.
- Eating at home is really important. So is making your food at home. This creates a feeling of loving intimacy with your body.
- If you're going to cook something lavish, like lasagne or a roast, enjoy, but eat smaller portions. Eat slowly and consider splitting your plate. Remember: It takes 15 min. to get the signal to your brain that you're full.
- Use olive oil instead of butter. Try new potatoes with artisan olive oil. If you're making mashed potatoes, use low fat buttermilk and low fat mayonnaise instead of butter and whole milk.
- If you're in a hurry, don't just grab fast food. Just think, what cooks quickly and easily? Fish, with a little salt and pepper and olive oil. Steam some vegetables, microwave some potatoes and you're done in minutes.
- Experiment with spices. Try dry rubs. Branch out.

Good eating and exercise go together. Work exercise into your life by being realistic about your lifestyle and true tolerance levels. As you work out, you discover how much your body craves good food—and your life begins to flow. Once you've cleared the pathway, your body will guide you to what it needs. Your body has wisdom. We've trained our bodies to shut up. But if you tune in, they'll speak to you.

Eating this way is a discipline, a very intimate discipline. In this chapter, I hope I've given you some of the tools you need to have your own healthy love affair with food.

A Few Words about Supplements

We have pollutants in our water, air and soils. Our soil is over-used. As a consequence, we're not getting the same nutrients we used to get from our food. We need some nutritional support. Here are some suggestions:

Multivitamins – Everybody should have a really good multi-vitamin. It's a relatively inexpensive way to support your efforts, a fortifying way to help insure that you're getting the nutrients you need to absorb food properly. This is doubly important if you work out. When you work out hard you create oxidation (free radicals). Anti-oxidants help to clean up those free radicals. As we've discussed, anti-oxidants come in the form of color: green and blue/purple, red, yellow and orange. In case you're not getting enough through your diet, help support your body with a multi-vitamin and a good antioxidant to help clean up free radicals. Usually everything you need doesn't come in a single tablet. There are some good companies out there. Do the research, make sure they're cold-processed, and find a good full-spectrum multivitamin in sufficient dosage. Critics will say we just pass multivitamins out in our urine, but that's true of the nutrients in everything. We absorb some and pass what we can't use.

Anti-aging supplements – Views about aging are changing a great deal these days. We're beginning to think of aging not as inevitability, but as a disease that can be successfully treated. There are some good resources to investigate, such as Antiaging-systems.com and Life Extension Foundation (www.LEF.org). These sites both sell supplements and have amazing research papers. One supplement to consider is **DHEA**, a testosterone precursor. One of the mistakes many doctors make, I believe, is that when women have problems with menopause, they prescribe estradiol or estrogen, but they don't supplement with testosterone. Find a doctor who will test your DHEA levels. Another is **Pregnenalone**. Considered the "mother hormone," it provides support for the hormone system as a whole. And to help you sleep, consider melatonin and tryptophan.

In short, you don't just have to accept some of the stressful aspects of aging. Do your research; educate yourself. Find an MD who specializes in anti-aging; that's a great way to go.

I've presented a lot of ideas here, but the idea isn't to overwhelm you or imply that you need to do everything. People who come to me often want to have giant breakthroughs all at once. But real change is modular. Let's change one thing at a time so it's not too overwhelming or confusing. Don't attempt too much at once, or you'll trip yourself up. You'll feel disappointed in yourself. You'll feel like a failure, it's a mad cycle. Start by changing small things. If you can go from buying frozen broccoli to fresh, and having your kids cut it up and steam it, good for you! That's one positive step!

Conclusion

AS I REFLECT BACK on why I undertook the project of writing this book, I see how much the journey has changed course. We struggled with how to encapsulate the contents into the perfect subtitle that would get the INTENT of the book through to you, the reader. I initially wanted to bring my bodybuilding TECHNIQUES to the average person, as well as the seasoned athlete. But in the course of writing this book over the last three years, I see how much more this project was than simply "that." It's about Bodybuilding as Art, Fitness and Spiritual Practice.

I realized all the personal revelations and insights that have come to me in the last 36 years of lifting weights, competing, learning and teaching, needed to somehow be woven together into a work that—hopefully—would inspire us all to EVOLVE past our own perceived limitations. I wanted to get you excited about the possibilities that connecting to your body can open up. This isn't "just" a book about getting the perfect physique. It's about taking control of who you are and who you can be, by plugging in to a more conscious way of being.

I want you to be excited to START. Once you see changes in your body, both appearance-wise as well as health-wise, you'll begin to feel better about so many things. And that's empowering!

With the conscious techniques laid out in this book, you can take weightlifting into your 80's, 90's and beyond. My goal is to live through those years as healthy, mobile and energetic as possible. And hopefully, still curious! I hope that you, too, can aspire to the same. You hold so much power in your hands. As I have learned – ANYTHING is possible. Had you asked me when I was 20 whether I could be a world champion bodybuilder, I would have said you were out of your mind. If you'd asked me when I was 30, if I could build four gyms, I'd have said you were insane. If you'd told me when I was 40 that one day I'd write a book, I would have never believed it possible. Most of the things I've done in my life, I would have never guessed would happen. So all I'm saying to you now is: DO. Don't over think it. Just start. And start again the next day. Start EVERY day, because the possibilities are endless.

> *Man often becomes what he believes himself to be. If I keep on saying to myself that I cannot do a certain thing, it is possible that I may end by really becoming incapable of doing it. On the contrary, if I have the belief that I can do it, I shall surely acquire the capacity to do it even if I may not have it at the beginning.*
>
> – Mahatma Gandhi

APPENDIX
What you Need to Know to Own your Workout

IN THIS APPENDIX:

- Why Gyms are Good—and a Good Personal Trainer is Great
- Choosing a Gym
- Gym Etiquette
- FAQs
- Other Tips & Pointers, including what you should know about injury

Why Gyms are Good—and a *Good* Personal Trainer is Great

First and foremost, I believe that everyone needs to get into a gym—a *good* gym that has the right atmosphere and a staff of good professional personal trainers.

You need a gym because you need to put yourself in a place focused on the single purpose of supporting you to become fit. This is especially true because our lives are so busy and fragmented. That's why many try to work out at home. But that is not likely to be as effective. Because you do so many other things there, it's full of potential distractions. Being in a gym, where the focus is on you and your fitness, switches on a different kind of energy, helping you to let go of distractions. Having a signal that helps you switch on a different kind of energy is really important. Here's a story to illustrate what I mean:

Before I started lifting weights, I tried running. One day, my doctor asked me what I was doing for exercise. I told him that I was running, but I hated it. My doctor, Scott Chilcott, who was himself a runner and bicyclist, gave me a tip that made all the difference. He suggested I buy a really good pair of running shoes and not to wear them unless I was going out to run. Don't use them for anything else, he said. That way, when you put them on, it sends a signal to your body-mind-spirit to let everything else fall away: you're going to *run* now. The same principle applies to a gym. Once you enter the gym, you're in a different mode. All the distractions are gone, and you can focus on your fitness.

How do I Choose a Gym?

The gym business has changed in recent years, and not necessarily for the better. There's pretty fierce competition between corporate-owned gyms and smaller, one-off enterprises. Unfortunately, when the "big box" gyms came along, they created a real change in the marketplace. They didn't seem as focused on fostering fitness as they were on marketing a product, and the "sells" were "hard." As a consequence, the experience felt a lot like buying used car, and people got in the habit of going to check out a gym with their armor up. You might have even made up your mind before you ever walked in: "I'm not going to buy a membership! I'm just here to look." You talked yourself out of joining because there was the fear of being taken for a ride, let alone the fear of not knowing how to use equipment, the fear of failure, etc., etc. So you told yourself you didn't want it anyway.

That's the culture that's been created around gyms.

So some gyms have massive marketing budgets, but are these the best gyms? Sometimes—but not always. Any gym will allow you to try it out for a small fee or for free, so go ahead. Just keep your wallet in the car until you're sure it's the gym for you. Here are some criteria to look for:

- You have to remember that a gym membership is an investment in yourself, first and foremost. Find a gym that makes you feel good about that investment.
- Find a *smart* gym. In most gyms, people don't get the understanding of their body and muscles that they really need. If you're new to gyms in general and don't have your internal focus already, you need support. Talk to the trainers to get a sense of their level of professionalism.
- What kind of programming do you want? What's going to get you pumped every day to get to the gym? Depending on what kinds of things you want to do for your fitness, check that the apppropriate equipment is there. Are there classes you want? If so, do they work for your time slots?
- Convenience - This is a key to increasing the likelihood of your showing up.
- Atmosphere - Look for a place where you feel comfortable, where you like the people who go there and the folks behind front desk are friendly, make you feel welcome and are likely to greet you by name when you check in.
- Cleanliness and order - It's impossible for everything in a public place to be spotless all the time, but a sense of cleanliness and order helps you feel good.

Do not buy based on price, but on services, feel and location.

Should I have a Personal Trainer?

Everyone new to the game should have a personal trainer, especially if you want to maximize your results and avoid injury. I know that a lot of us think we can just do it ourselves, but it's like picking up a golf club and thinking you can play golf right away, without a single lesson. Or thinking you can just start playing the piano. You can't. In fact, we get lots of injuries in gyms because people don't know what they're doing. Getting fit is an investment in yourself, and you need to think of it that way. You want this discipline and modality around for the rest of your life. You need to get launched, so get help, especially at the beginning. It's available, and it's not expensive, especially when you consider how much money we freely spend on things that don't benefit our health so much: snack food, alcohol and coffee out, movie and concert tickets, internet and cable television, etc. Put those things aside for a month or two and save your money for personal trainer. That doesn't mean you have to have a personal trainer every time you go to a weight room.

A good trainer is a teacher—not just a cheerleader. They're there to teach you, not just to push you through exercises. It's about having a partner who makes sure you develop good habits from the very beginning.

What should I look for in a Personal Trainer?

Here are my suggestions for the top seven criteria to use when choosing a trainer:

1. **Experience** – Time in the business is a big factor to consider. There are a lot of young personal trainers out there, but how qualified are they, really? In the past becoming a trainer was more experiential; now it's more cerebral. Would you be comfortable with a surgeon who'd never operated before? You want a trainer who is capable of tuning into *you* versus taking a rote approach. That only comes with experience. So, look for experience of a certain kind.
2. **A Good Role Model** - Look for what they've done with their own physique. Do they look like they know what they're doing? Every trainer doesn't have to be former bodybuilder or an ex-

treme athlete, but they should be good examples for you; they should look trim and fit and healthy. That said, I have a trainer on staff who is 90 lbs. overweight—but she's very fit. She's lost 100 lbs., so she's a great example to others. Plus, she's got one of the best eyes around. She can watch you exercise and know immediately if something's not right, and help you fix it. She reminds us all that it's not about having a Barbie body, but about being the best that your personal capacity will allow.

3. **Interested in You** - So much of the job of being a personal trainer lies in discovering where people are coming from, *i.e.*, what motivates them and what their resistances are. A good trainer should gather information about you on a number of levels, if you're willing to give it. I want to know how you can fit fitness into your lifestyle, so I ask a lot of questions at the beginning. For example, if I'm training a 35-yr-old woman with several kids at home, she will have challenges different from those of a single woman. It also helps if they're intuitive. Your body is such an intimate tool; everything we've ever experienced has come to us through this body. The trainer's job is to take all that in and work with it. I find I have to be a bit of both an empath and shapeshifter. I have to climb into my client's body to understand why he or she moves that way. If I get stymied, then I'm going to do some research until I come up with an answer for my client.
4. **Easy to Relate to** – Despite television programs like *The Biggest Loser,* your trainer should not intimidate you. You should feel that they're able to tune into you and your particular challenges. For example, even though I don't have a weight problem, I had to take my body down to 6% body fat when I was competing, so I do know what it's like to diet. I know what it's like to crave foods, and to want to quit.
5. **Takes Hands-On Approach** – Your trainer should be willing to show you, not just tell you. They should watch you and help you

make corrections or adjustments rather than just taking you through a series of exercises.

6. **Displays an Open Attitude and Willingness to Learn** – Good trainers are always learning and willing to learn. I didn't grow up in world of "functional training," but I watch what they do, and learn. Your trainer should be open and always bringing you new ideas and options. They should be willing to confer with your doctor and refer you to one if you need it. Many trainers don't refer often enough. Sometimes talking to a doctor can open up a whole new vista.
7. **Is Available to You** – Once you hire a trainer, you should feel they've taken you on as a project. For example, do they text you to ask how you're doing today after workout? Or send you a daily reminder, such as: "Hey, today, how about doing a vigorous walk and 20 push- ups?" Or, "Today, try to eat not more than 1500 calories." These kinds of things show they're invested in your success.

Remember, you don't need to commit to one trainer. Before you buy a package, shop around and try different people. First observe how they work. Buy at least one session with a trainer first. See how well you get along. Chemistry is big deal. Make your decision based on your personal experience with them.

This comes back to making the most of your time in the gym. If you go in there and you don't know how to work out and you just start fumbling around, maybe you'll hit on something, maybe you won't. You will need a guide, and you should budget for it. A good personal trainer is worth the money, as my clients can attest.

Gym Etiquette - or - How Not to Look Like a Rookie

Many times I find that even people who have been around gyms for years have somehow missed out on understanding the basics. These fundamentals represent the foundation upon which you build. When you don't have these, you're not building on solid ground, and one day it's bound to catch up to you. Lack of knowledge can make you feel uncomfortable, and we don't want people to feel uncomfortable.

So, yes, gyms have a special etiquette that people need to understand. In this section I'll go over some of these basics. If you find you know them all already, just take a moment to review them. If they're new to you, then take a moment each day or week to review until they're part of your repertoire.

Catt's Ten (or So) Gym Commandments:

1. Dress properly - No "street" clothes, boots or jeans.
2. Keep the workout area uncluttered - Keep your gym bags and magazines off the workout floor. Clear your bench.
3. Respect all gym equipment - Dropping weights is an absolute no-no.
4. Return equipment to its proper place after use; there's a reason you can find what you need when you walk in. For example, if you put weights on a machine—or if they're already there—take a moment when you finish to remove them and put them back on the proper storage rack. Weight racks are generally organized by 5-, 10-, 25-, 35- and 45-lbs. Don't lean plates against the wall or the machines.
5. Be aware of your surroundings and respect the people there! Be considerate of others by being aware of who is using what. If someone is using a mirror to check his or her form, don't stand in the way, for example. Likewise, don't talk to someone when they're in the middle of a set.
6. Share - If someone says, "May I work in with you," say "Yes." Likewise, if you work in with someone, be prompt.
7. Watch your personal noise level - Grunting and screaming are distracting to others. They're also not helpful to you, as you're

expending energy out rather than conserving it and using it to lift the weight.

8. Cell phones - Shut off the ring tone, and do not answer your cell phone unless you're a doctor or a parent responding to an emergency.
9. No swearing - No abusive language. Honestly, no one wants to hear it.
10. Smells - The gym is not the place for perfumes and colognes. And, for goodness sake, please wear clean clothes and shower!
11. Use the collars on the bars to hold the weights on - A lot of folks (you know who you are) resist putting collars on bars; they think it's a sissy thing. But it's not. The collar actually holds the weights on so they don't come off. When they do, people can get hurt. Some people don't put them on because they're trying to lift a heavier weight for the first time, and they think they might need to be able to dump the weights off if they can't do it. No! The action of the weights dropping off is so violent that you won't be able to control the bar—and that can lead to tearing a muscle. If you're trying to move a new, heavier weight for the first time, definitely **put the collars on** and ask to work with a good spotter who can help you.

FAQs

Q: Should I have a Training Partner?

A: This is not a "yes" or "no" question because a training partner can be either very beneficial or detrimental. A training partner can be beneficial because you can help support each other to sign up for a gym and go regularly. For many women, this is almost an imperative. But I say "detrimental" because the minute you add another person to the mix, you add another variable that's out of your control. If that person wants to do something different from what you want to do that can sometimes be good, but it can also be bad. If they don't match you on energetic level, they can drag you down to theirs, etc. And if your training partner moves away, then what happens? The point is: always rely on yourself first. You have to find it within yourself to train, whether alone or with someone. *You* are the constant. You're the one who always has to show up.

Here are some things to look for in a training partner. You want someone who:

- Will motivate you, if that's what you need.
- Matches you closely, strength-wise, or at least is willing to accommodate your strength capacities
- Has the same motivations and time frames as you do.
- Shows up consistently

A person who fits all these criteria is difficult to find. With only one exception, I could never find a training partner who didn't pull me away mentally from my workout. If you find a great training partner, that's awesome. But don't rely on someone else. Learn to train by yourself no matter what because it's really about making a connection with yourself.

Q: Heavy or Light?

A: With respect to weights, people ask me all the time, should I go heavy or light?

First of all, "heavy" or "light" are relative terms. It's all in the mind. Your mind may tell you that "heavy" means 300 lbs., but that's just a number. If a weight is tough to pull correctly, then that's heavy—for you. People I've worked with tell me all the time that I can make 10 pounds feel like 100. That's true, because it's not just the number on the weight you're lifting, it's *how* you're lifting it. Now that you understand my technique you can see why that's so.

There are also different advantages to lifting heavy and lifting light, as the research shows. Research tells us that when we lift "heavy," (as you might do in compound motions, such as squats, dead lifts, bench press, pull ups, dips, etc.,) that because of the sheer amount of muscle incorporated to do those lifts, growth hormone output is naturally increased.[86] (http://www.ncbi.nlm.nih.gov/pubmed/15831061)

Testosterone increases as well, with weight training. These are hormones that decline as we age. So if we have a way of increasing our body's output of those things, why wouldn't we do that?

Q: What's One of the Most Common Mistakes People Make?

A. People don't use proper shoes when they're lifting. They wear running shoes with a big, thick, soft sole. These shoes are meant for cushioning the impact and providing a little bounce when your foot hits the ground or pavement. They're great for running, but they provide the absolute worst foot position for lifting weights. Think about it: A 200 lb. guy squatting 300 lbs. means he's putting 500 lbs. on a pair of running shoes. It's like squatting on a waterbed! There's no stability for your knees and there's constant reverberation from foot to ankle to knee to hip and back, because it's a soft heel. On top that, these shoes pitch you forward. When you lift, you want to feel as much of your foot as flat as possible, connected with the ground. When I lift—with proper shoes—I visualize the top of my foot coming up, the balls of my feet pressing down. Got knee problems? Get out of those running shoes!

Q: How Much Should I work out?

A: As a general rule for bodybuilding, do at least 3-5 exercises in each workout, with at least three sets of each exercise per body part. In general, that means 9-15 sets/day per body part. But these rules can drift. Once you learn to tune into your body, you'll know what you need on any particular day. Remember: More is not always better. For example, if I feel particularly good on a given day, I may do 6 or 7 sets of a certain exercise. It just depends. Listen to your body.

Q: When should I work out?

A: Tuning in to your body's natural rhythms is part of getting to know yourself. When does your body want to work out?

For example, I'm not a morning person; so going to the gym at 5 AM is just not for me. I love the energy of the 5 PM crowd. I love a noisy, crowded gym filled with people I know and love. There's a little of the peacock in me. I feed on that energy; it reinforces the idea that I'm doing something worthy. It's fun to be a woman pushing a lot of weight and to have people noticing that. It's fun to have that gym camaraderie. We have a good time out there. If I'm out there by myself, I don't have as good a time. When I'm in my set, I'm focused, but in between sets, when I'm stretching or whatever, I'm joking, etc. I have a good time. I think that social aspect is what keeps people coming back to the gym. This is a community.

I've noticed, though, that those who work out first thing in the morning are more likely to keep it up. If you plan your workout for later in the day, chances are you'll have lots of other things pulling at you. But if it's your first move of the day, it's done.

Find your own body's rhythms. Some have to force themselves into a rhythm because of life circumstances, which is understandable, but it's better if you just try some different things and watch for what seems to work best. You'll probably find you have to make some compromises. If you like 5 PM, but you find too many distractions, you need to switch to a time that works better for you, whether your body wants to or not.

Q: How often should I work out?

A: You might expect me to say as often as possible, but I know that some of us have a tendency to go to extremes and overdo it. One of the biggest pitfalls of a newbie is the tendency to over-commit.

You absolutely *don't* have to be in the gym every day. But that said, I try to do something physical daily. Maybe it's mountain biking or just walking the golf course or maybe it's yoga. And remember that you need downtime to recover, re-build and repair. You also need good food to help you recover and repair. Give yourself those things.

If you're going to work out after work, keep your gym bag in the car. Don't go home, because if you do, too many other things can happen. Always have your gym bag packed and ready to go. If you're on the road, try to keep the habit, even if you get in just a couple of workouts.

Expert Tips & Pointers

Here are some pointers for how to stay safe and avoid injury.

1. Exercise Basics: By the Numbers

It's important to understand the difference between exercises, sets, and reps.

- An exercise is a specific movement for a specific purpose. For example, the bench press is an exercise to develop the chest muscles.
- A "rep" stands for repetition. It means one performance of a single movement. In general, we benefit from repeating the movement several times. For example, if I do a specific movement ten times, that equals "ten reps."
- A set, then, is composed of a series of one or more reps, performed continuously, ending with a rest period. For Example: one set may consist of three, five, or ten or more reps, depending upon what's right for your body at any given time.

2. The Importance of Feedback

Why are there mirrors in gyms? Most people probably think it's about "ego tripping," but it's not. (OK, maybe sometimes!) But the true reason is that mirrors are fabulous feedback mechanisms, and feedback is essential when you're trying to learn something new.

I always direct people to observe their body in the mirror. I want to help them get beyond the superficial view, which can often involve negative judgments, and see the underlying structure of their physique. It's part of developing that intimate connection with their body that I discussed earlier.

The mirror is also a great learning tool. It helps you learn new patterns of movement. When I get people moving in a new way, and I'll have them watch themselves in the mirror. Getting it visually is the first step.

When you connect what you're seeing with what you're feeling, you create a new imprint. So I have them close their eyes and duplicate the movement. "Close your eyes and see it on the inside," I'll say. They start to make a connection between what they know they should look like and what that feels like in their body.

This is especially important if someone's been in a negative pattern for a long time. You'd be surprised how many times people don't tell me about issues with their bodies. They've lived with some of these things for so long that it just feels normal to them. For example, I've worked with people who have scoliosis, but didn't tell me. Then I'll have them move, and I'll see it. In cases like these, imprinting through both sight and feeling is critical—and mirrors provide a vital form of feedback for them.

3. How to Work with a Spotter

Use a spotter when you want to attempt to lift a weight you haven't done before or don't feel confident with. So the first criterion for choosing a spotter is to find someone who's capable of doing what you're trying to do. But that said, a spotter's role is to assist you gently, to keep the bar moving. It's not to take the full weight. If you're failing, your spotter should never have to hold the whole the thing up. *Never.*

That goes along with another general rule, which is: *Do not overreach*. And that's connected to another rule: *Always be in control of the weight*. Frequently, I observe guys thinking they're capable of doing more than they really can, so their spotters end up helping from first rep to last. That's not acceptable; it's not what a spot is about. I will not spot someone who doesn't know what they're doing. If I have to save you, you shouldn't be doing it in the first place.

If you're asked to spot, be discriminating. If someone with 315 lbs. on the bar asks you to spot for them, evaluate the situation. If you have *any doubts* about your ability to pull up 315 pounds, please feel free to say, "No, I'm not comfortable spotting you. " Don't put yourself—or the other person—in jeopardy, especially out of pride. It happens all the time, and it can be dangerous.

There's a technique to giving good spot. You want to keep weight moving. If the person you're spotting for still wants to stay with it and struggle, don't lift the weight out of their hands. Help them complete the lift with the appropriate amount of effort.

Look around your gym and find out who the best spotters are. Find out who's a real resource and who to never to ask again. Finding a good spotter can be a process of trial and error.

4. How to Stay Safe

When it comes to safety, one of the most important things you need to know is where and how to "bail-out."

In brief, you need a predetermined plan for how you'll safely get out of an exercise if you need to. If you're pulling a cable, there's not much to worry about, but with free weights, you need a bailout plan. If, for example, you're attempting to bench press a new weight—and you don't have a spotter—you absolutely need to know what your bailout plan is.

You can't be fully present in your workout if you feel unsafe or unfamiliar. This can be especially true for those who are not used to lifting weights. If you're doing a lift for the first time and your mind/body registers it as heavy, and it's coming at you, you can panic. Then you can begin struggling and twisting; when you can't hold your form, that's when injuries happen. To counteract that, I teach people how to plan their bailouts.

Here's a rule of thumb: *If you can't come back up with that bar, come down.*

So always look first to familiarize yourself with the situation and determine where your bailouts are. Typically, if you're doing a bench press, there's a rack where the weight sits and then two more prongs below. So if you get all the way down and realize you can't come up all the way, usually you can come up a little bit and put it back on the lower rung. The same thing goes for squats. There are what we call bail out racks.

When people are new to weightlifting, I always take them through a process to help them get familiar with their bailouts. I have them bring the weight as low as they can and feel the safety stops. Then I'll put some more weight on and have them practice while I'm watching so they can see that the weight won't fall on them. They need to feel that sense of confidence, get it into your body and brain, so they know they can bail out if they need to.

Remember; always do what's right for YOU, because we want you safe and back in the gym.

5. What you should know about Injury

When I work with people I ask whether they've had any injuries before we start. Then we'll start to work, and as I watch them move, I'll see something they haven't mentioned. "What's going on?" I'll ask. "Did you have a back injury?" Very often they'll respond, "Oh, yeah, but it's healed." Well, that's not completely true because I saw it. The injury may have healed in one sense, but it's still being held in their body.

I think this happens because the body is so fast to adapt to injury; it does so by compensating. This happens outside of our awareness. We tend to want to protect any area that's received any kind of injury—so we'll shorten our range of motion, or we'll "favor" one side over the other, which means one side is bearing more weight than the other. This redistribution may seem like a subtle adjustment at the time, but it has lasting repercussions.

We get protective around injuries and we end up doing more damage in the long run because we haven't paid conscious attention to balance, symmetry, etc., as we're healing from an injury. So, typically, there's a cascade effect: the cure for an injury creates problems elsewhere. Here's an example: If someone injures their left foot, they're told to wear a hard shoe on that foot alone. While this helps stabilize their injured foot, they also begin walking in an unbalanced way. Then, later, they wonder why they have back problems. If we have some awareness of how this might affect our body as a whole, we could do some corrective exercises along the way to make sure there's no further damage being done.

Here's another example of how an injury—and the cure for an injury—might adversely affect the whole. Years ago, I had a friend who lost limb, and then was given an artificial limb. There was a difference in weight between his actual arm and the prosthetic, but because that was never attended to, it led to a gradual twisting of his spine. There was an asymmetry. This happens even on the micro scale. If you wear a cast on your right arm, especially with a sling, for eight weeks, that's not what your body is used to. It'll cause problems in other areas.

Life is not injury-free. I know from first-hand experience; I've been in two major car accidents. Most people think they have to stop everything if they get an injury. No. When you get an injury, the worst thing you can do is leave it alone, let it atrophy and freeze; ideally, you want to keep it moving. If you stop working out because you've sustained an injury, you can actually make the situation worse. You're creating more weakness around that injury. The beauty of strength training is that you can start consciously to build things back up—to the degree that you can, given the state of the body. This is always going to be better than leaving it alone.

Remember that old joke: "Doc, it hurts when I do this." "Well," says the doc, "Don't do that." We still have doctors who'll tell you not to do anything when you're injured. (I actually had a client with a minor hemorrhoid, whose doctor suggested stopping his weight training altogether, as a cure! Really?) They're finally figuring out that "bad backs," for example, do not benefit from rest. I've been talking about this for 15-20 years!

In my mind, the medical community is maybe ten years behind people like me in certain, limited circumstances, because we're willing to experiment on ourselves. And we notice things. We may not have the papers, the medical proof, the double-blind studies, but there are things that I know. I know it's not good for me to sit and not move. My body craves movement. Everybody's body does. At least now with knee and hip replacements, when they're doing ACL's and things like that, they get you moving the next day. This is all relatively new.

Working around injury

There's *almost always* a way around of injury. It just may take some investigation and some adjustments. Of course, some injuries are impossible to work around. I'm not going to expect someone to do leg presses or squats if they've just had an ACL repair in the last week—but there are always some exercises that you can do. Leaving it alone is never the best thing to do. Even moving it in slightest way helps you re-invigorate, gets the blood pumping to area, etc., so you don't lose those connections. This is where strength training is such a boon, as is having a trainer who knows how to work with you and your injury.

As an example, one time I was doing a triceps exercise. For some reason, I got distracted—something pulled my attention away—and I slightly strained a tendon. I could no longer do the exercise I was doing for triceps, at least on that angle. I knew if I pushed it, the whole thing could give way. It was that bad. I immediately tried to find some other exercise for triceps that I could do. But light or heavy, I just couldn't do it, and that really bothered me.

So little by little over the next several weeks, I looked for something I could do. And it got better over the week. I still had to baby it and work around it but I got a decent triceps workout in. It wasn't epic, but it was decent. And with each successive week, it healed a little more. I never stopped trying to work it, but I did pay attention to my body. Each time I tried, I sensed that this angle or this way I'm doing the exercise needed to shift, even slightly. I kept trying to exercise it, and simultaneously, it progressively got better. Two months later, I could still feel traces of the injury, but I was doing all the things I was doing before. Eventually, it went away entirely.

Periodically, things will just happen, and you'll need to learn to work around those injuries/vulnerabilities. Just don't stop—if that's possible. It's not always possible, but it very often is. And if you can't figure out how yourself, check in a knowledgeable trainer. Not all trainers know how, so find one who does.

If you're contemplating a joint replacement

One day, one of our members, who had been really working hard, didn't show up for his "leg day." When I asked him why, he said his doctor told him not to because he was a candidate for knee replacement.

OK, listen up, because I'm going to disagree strongly. Having more muscle tissue—rather than less—is always a good thing. Any time you allow a muscle to atrophy, you're creating a potential disaster. There are some amazing things being done with knee replacements now, but you want to be as strong as you possibly can be before you go into surgery.

If you're in the process of deciding whether to get a knee or hip replacement, please consider the following:

- Buy as much time as you can. How much longer can you manage, without creating problems anywhere else in the body? Because medical science advances so quickly, the difference between waiting one year or five for surgery can make an enormous difference. For example, now they have gender-specific replacement knees. They couldn't understand why they were getting more failures of artificial knees in women until they realized that the configuration of female knees is different enough to require a gender-specific knee.
- Lose some weight, because your weight makes such a difference. Extra weight takes a huge toll on our knees. It's no coincidence that many people with knee or hip problems tend to be heavy.
- If you're able to walk, there are things a personal trainer like me can do with you to strengthen your leg so it will hold the joint together better. The stronger you are before surgery, the shorter your recovery time.

NOTES

1. http://www.etymonline.com/index.php?term=health
2. http://www.sparrowdancer.com/perception.html
3. http://www.shareable.net/blog/birds-do-it-bats-do-it
4. http://bioteaching.wordpress.com/2010/10/15/the-evolution-of-cooperation/
5. Tu Moonwalker was a spiritual teacher and minister. In 1988, she founded with her sister Láne Saán, the Philosophy of Universal Beingness within the Whole, a spiritual system based on environmental consciousness and peaceful coexistence. Born of Apache and South American Native American parents, Tu was raised on the White Mountain Apache reservations in Arizona. Tu's accomplishments were many. Academically, she held undergraduate degrees in Anthropology and Biochemistry and graduate degrees in Museum Science and Geology. Musically gifted, she collaborated on the lyrics for "Puff the Magic Dragon" and "Dust in the Wind." Her book, *Business Revolution through Ancestral Wisdom* (Outskirts Press, 2008) received the 2009 New Mexico Book Award in Business. Tu was an accomplished artisan, and her artwork is in several private and museum collections, including the Smithsonian Institution.
6. *From Paradise Lost to Paradise Regained* by Watchtower Society (Jehovah's Witnesses, 1st ed., 1958).
7. http://health.howstuffworks.com/human-body/parts/16-unusual-facts-about-the-human-body10.htm
8. http://icantseeyou.typepad.com/my_weblog/2008/02/100-very-cool-f.html
9. Sources for amazing facts about human body: http://listverse.com/2008/06/10/top-15-amazing-facts-about-the-human-body/
10. http://voices.yahoo.com/the-human-body-10-most-amazing-things-can-5464321.html?cat=58

11. http://www.wiziq.com/tutorial/39073-Explore-the-human-body-your-amazing-machine
12. http://www.cafeoflifepikespeak.com/amazing_facts.htm
13. *The Future of the Body: Explorations Into the Further Evolution Of Human Nature* by Michael Murphy (TarcherPerigree, 1993).
14. http://www.ted.com/talks/juan_enriquez_will_our_kids_be_a_different_species.html
15. "Expert performance: Its structure and acquisition" by Ericsson, K. Anders; Charness, Neil. American Psychologist, Vol 49(8), Aug 1994, 725-747.
16. https://www.ted.com/talks/juan_enriquez_will_our_kids_be_a_different_species?language=en
17. Say you're born without a limb. Well, that may be a real limitation that you'll have to accept—but it's also true that lizards and salamanders can regenerate lost limbs. If these creatures can re-grow body parts, then why not humans? Perhaps the potential is there, and we just haven't learned how to tap it yet. In fact, researchers are already working on regenerating human teeth from stem cells (see: http://www.wndu.com/mmm/headlines/151166685.html). Researchers are also inquiring into the mechanisms that underlie an animal's ability to regenerate. Tadpoles, for example, can regenerate their tails because of a natural process that alters the electrical properties of their cells. The build-up of electrical charge at the site of amputation then seems to help guide tissue regeneration. Scientists have known for some time that applied electrical fields can influence tissue growth, but exactly how the body itself produces electrical fields to promote tissue regeneration remained a mystery. With further research of this kind, doctors might one day be able to regenerate tissue in patients - such as those who have suffered spinal cord injury - by applying electrical charges to alter the flow of positively charged molecules out of cells. (See: http://www.newscientist.com/article/dn11273-electrical-tweaking-helps-tadpole-grow-new-tail.html).
18. Source: Early release of selected estimates based on data from the 2011 National Health Interview Survey, data tables for figures 7.1, 8.1, 9.1
19. http://www.rejuvinstitute.com/blog/health/children%E2%80%99s-nutrition-statistics-reflect-scary-truths/#.UOzEl7ZyWw8
20. http://healthy-living.org/html/what_a_choice_.html

21. http://www.drugabuse.gov/publications/topics-in-brief/prescription-drug-abuse
22. http://www.drugabuse.gov/related-topics/trends-statistics
23. Read more: http://www.livestrong.com/article/329044-exercises-for-ligaments-tendons/#ixzz259dW3Mw9
24. Ligaments and tendons are also trainable. According to the Muscle and Strength website, training, increasing their thickness, strength and stiffness by up to 20 percent. Strengthening your ligaments and tendons has benefits: it can decrease your risk of injury so that you avoid long recovery periods, as well as the need for medication or even surgery.
25. http://www.drmirkin.com/public/ezine100211.html
    http://www.futurepundit.com/archives/008296.html
    http://well.blogs.nytimes.com/2011/09/28/how-exercise-can-strengthen-the-brain/
    http://www.news-medical.net/news/20110920/Regular-exercise-also-increases-mitochondrial-numbers-in-brain-cells.aspx
26. Reporting in Cell Metabolism, researchers write that when people who lead relatively sedentary lives worked out, the DNA in their muscle fibers changed almost immediately. http://www.npr.org/2012/03/09/148306989/a-workout-can-change-your-dna and http://healthland.time.com/2012/03/07/how-exercise-can-change-your-dna/
27. http://longevity.about.com/od/lifelongfitness/a/exercise_energy.htm
28. http://blog.focusedtrainers.com/2010/10/01/how-does-exercise-increase-energy/
    http://www.bettermovement.org/2012/fatigue-is-an-emotion/
29. http://www.sciencedaily.com/releases/2006/11/061101151005.htm
    http://www.webmd.com/diet/news/20061103/exercise-fights-fatigue-boosts-energy
    http://www.mayoclinic.com/health/exercise/HQ01676
    http://www.sharecare.com/question/how-does-exercise-improve-energy
    http://www.livestrong.com/article/401475-does-blood-flow-to- the-brain-increase-during-exercise/
30. http://well.blogs.nytimes.com/2009/11/18/phys-ed-why-exercise-makes-you-less-anxious/

31. See http://www.scientificamerican.com/article/how-to-grow-stronger-without-lifting-weights/
32. http://cepuk.org/2014/04/30/council-evidence-based-psychiatry-launches-today-data-showing-dramatic-rise-mental-health-disability/
33. Paul Hawken, commencement speech, 2009 http://www.yesmagazine.org/issues/columns/you-are-brilliant-and-the-earth-is-hiring
34. See: http://www.scientificamerican.com/article.cfm?id=ultimate-social-network-bacteria-protects-health
35. Read more: http://www.umm.edu/altmed/articles/spirituality-000360.htm#ixzz2A9rGvqiK
36. See *The Evolutionaries: Unlocking the Spiritual and Cultural Potential of Science's Greatest Idea* by Carter Phipps (Harper Perennial, 2012), p. 329.
37. http://www.liveyourlifept.com/blog/2014/08/19/middle-age-spread-weight-gain-help/
38. Read more: http://www.livestrong.com/artcle/452842-strength-training-for-women-over-60-years-old/#ixzz2ixATrTR9
39. "The Health Benefits Of Weightlifting And The New Science That Supports Strength Building," by Julie Wilcox, published in Forbes, 5/31/2012.
40. "Create Your Best Body for Aging" by Tim Bean posted on the website http:www.antiaging-systems.com: http://www.antiaging-systems.com/articles/341-create-your-best-body-for-aging?utm_medium=email&utm_campaign=Bean and Laing article, sermorelin, ghrp2, dep pro, 1st line, d3&utm_source=YMExpress
41. http://io9.gizmodo.com/5953154/why-getting-physically-stronger-will-help-you-to-live-longer
42. http://skylertanner.com/2012/04/15/finally-strength-training-and-its-effects-on-the-biomarkers-of-aging/
43. http://www.dukehealth.org/health_library/health_articles/the-unquestionable-benefits-of-strength-training
44. http://www.forbes.com/sites/juliewilcox/2012/05/31/health-benefits-weightlifting/
45. http://www.restartretirement.com/2013/04/08/strength-training-older-adults/
46. http://io9.gizmodo.com/5953154/why-getting-physically-stronger-will-help-you-to-live-longer

47. Growth hormone is produced by the pituitary gland in the brain and stimulates the growth of muscle, cartilage, and bone. It stimulates growth in children and plays an important role in adult metabolism. It is made throughout a person's lifetime but declines with age. See also: http://nstarzone.com/EXERCISE.html
48. http://www.sentientdevelopments.com/2013/01/why-getting-physically-stronger-will.html
49. 5953154/why-getting-physically-stronger-will-help-you-to-live-longer
50. http://breakingmuscle.com/health-medicine/growth-hormone-how-does-it-work-and-why-do-women-have-more; http://breakingmuscle.com/health-medicine/what-women-need-to-know-about-growth-hormone-and-how-to-maximize-it
51. See for example: http://www.crossfittt.com/will-lifting-heavy-weights-make-me-big/
52. Note: This is very different from power lifting, which involves a burst of energy, but does not work with your pain threshold in quite the same way.
53. For more on EMDR see: http://www.emdr.com/
54. Weider went so far as to talk about a "muscle confusion" principle, but no one's broken this concept down the way I have; he never brought in the body-mind-spirit connection.
55. http://www.emdr.com/history-of-emdr/
56. http://www.nejm.org/doi/full/10.1056/NEJMoa1200303?query=featured_home&&, http://www.thedailybeast.com/articles/2013/02/27/eat-like-a-greek-themediterranean-diet-that-could-save-your-life.html
57. http://healthyeating.sfgate.com/average-calorie-intake-human-per-day-versus-recommendation-1867.html
58. http://naturalsociety.com/average-american-diet-infographic/
59. Read more: http://www.livestrong.com/article/347737-the-average-american-daily-caloric-intake/#ixzz2NRkAe9me
60. A 2.4oz portion of french fries has grown to 6.7oz; hamburgers from 3.9oz to 12oz; and soda from 7oz to 42oz. See reference below.
61. Read more: http://naturalsociety.com/portion-sizes-restaurants-quadruple/#ixzz2LYqa2we4
62. http://www.naturalworldhealing.com/Dentalinfo/food-toxin-dangers.htm

63. http://thechart.blogs.cnn.com/2010/06/25/a-tale-of-2-nuggets/ http://en.wikipedia.org/wiki/Polydimethylsiloxane
64. http://farmwars.info/?p=4897
65. http://www.takepart.com/node/34851
66. http://www.cdc.gov/chronicdisease/resources/publications/aag/ chronic.htm
67. http://www.takepart.com/node/34851
68. http://www.diabetes.org/diabetes-basics/statistics/?referrer=https:// www.google.com/
69. http://www.emory.edu/policysolutions/chronic_disease.html
70. (http://www.nybooks.com/articles/archives/2010/jun/10/food-movement-rising/?pagination=false
71. http://www.nytimes.com/2013/02/24/magazine/the-extraordinary-science-of-junk-food.html?ref=magazine&_r=2&
72. http://thinkprogress.org/health/2012/07/26/589041/crop-subsidies-obesity/?mobile=nc
73. http://cornsubsidies.com/
74. http://www.takepart.com/article/2013/03/12/when-good-food-goes-bad-americans-pay-price
75. http://www.gracelinks.org/265/environment
76. http://www.nybooks.com/articles/archives/2010/jun/10/food-movement-rising/?pagination=false
77. See: *The Shaman Within: A Physcist's Guide to the Deeper Dimensions of Your Life, the Universe, Everything by Claude Poncelet* (Sounds True, 2014)
78. http://www.super-lutein.net/en/gl/faq.html
79. http://health.howstuffworks.com/wellness/food-nutrition/vitamin-supplements/what-are-carotenoids.htm
80. http://www.phytochemicals.info/antioxidants.php
81. Adapted from:http://www.foodinsight.org/Newsletter/Detail.aspx?topic= Eat_a_Rainbow_Functional_Foods_and_Their_Colorful_Components and http://www.wholeliving.com/
82. http://lpi.oregonstate.edu/infocenter/phytochemicals/resveratrol/
83. Research on Flavanoids: http://www.news-medical.net/health/ What-are-Flavonoids.aspx and http://lpi.oregonstate.edu/infocenter/ phytochemicals/flavonoids/

84. http://www.phytochemicals.info/phytochemical-tips.php
85. http://saferchemicals.org/newsroom/12949/
86. http://www.ncbi.nlm.nih.gov/pubmed/15831061

how did you know
that you were meant
to be a healer?

because i kept
falling in love
with broken people.

then why
are you alone?

because i'm broken too
so i am falling
in love with myself
to get a taste
of my own medicine

–kwabena foli

ABOUT THE AUTHOR

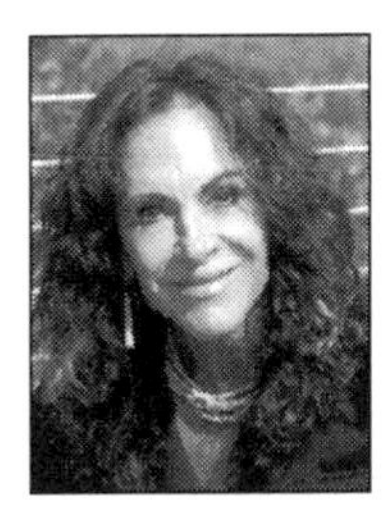

CATT TRIPOLI, also known as **Cathey Palyo,** is a former professional bodybuilder who has been involved in the health and fitness field for over 30 years. She has been the creative force behind four gyms, including Powerhouse Gym in Santa Rosa, CA, which she currently owns and operates.

Bodybuilding saved Catt's life; through dedicated practice, she gained not only outer strength, but an inner resilience that transcends sport.

Raised in an apocryphal religious belief system that severely restricted both aspirations and involvement with the outside world, Catt found the courage to break away and seek her own path. Once she found bodybuilding, she rose quickly through the amateur ranks, earning her pro card by winning the overall title at the Ms. Universe competition in Singapore in 1986. In 1988 she won the Ms. International contest (now the Arnold Classic), the highlight of her professional bodybuilding career. She has been featured on the covers of *Muscular Development* and *Muscle & Fitness* magazines, as well as several international fitness publications in Belgium, France, Mexico, the Netherlands, and Greece. She was only the second woman to be featured on the cover of *Flex*, bodybuilding's premier magazine.

Catt is available for both fitness training and hypnotherapy, and can be reached at **Catt.consciousfitness@gmail.com**.

Made in the USA
Middletown, DE
21 October 2016